Teen Girl's Handbook

Book 1

FIND YOUR CONFIDENCE

BEAT STRESS, MAKE REAL FRIENDS

AND LOVE WHO YOU ARE

Teenskill Surge

Contents

A Note from the Author

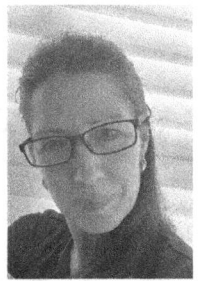

Hi, I'm Monika, the author behind *Teen Girl's Handbook*.

As I embarked on creating this book, I drew on my own experiences. I remember the challenges of balancing friendships, school, and self-confidence, and the overwhelming feelings that often accompanied these struggles. I wanted to create a haven for every girl who has ever felt not good enough, left out, or unsure of where she fits.

This book was written to remind you that you don't have to have it all figured out to grow. You don't have to be perfect to be worthy of love, friendship, or peace. You can start exactly where you are—one small, honest step at a time.

Every page in this handbook is a treasure trove of practical tools for confidence, calm, and connection. I hope that as you read, you'll come to see yourself not as someone who needs fixing, but as someone who is already becoming everything she's meant to be.

I am deeply grateful for the opportunity to be part of your journey. These words will serve as a beacon of courage when things feel hard, and a gentle reminder that you are never walking alone.

With gratitude and encouragement,

— Monika

For updates, encouragement, and new releases, scan the QR code below to follow **MM Legacy Publishing** on Facebook for helpful resources and upcoming books from both the **TeenSkill Surge** and **Graceful Growth** collections.

READER BONUS

BONUS #1 – TEEN GIRL'S HANDBOOK COMPANION

Access your free journal to start building confidence and calm today!

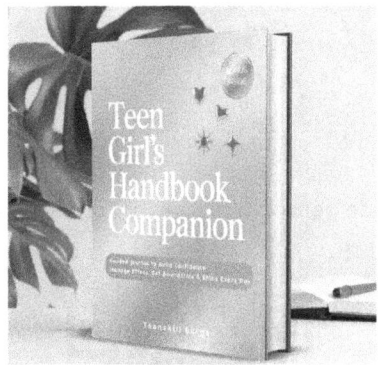

Scan the QR code to download your bonus guide!
Start exploring right away — it's yours to keep and enjoy.

***

BONUS #2 – TEEN GIRL'S HANDBOOK, BOOK 2

Continue your growth journey with Book 2—
confidence, purpose, and resilience await!

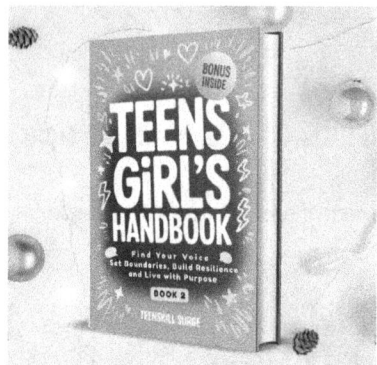

Simply scan the QR code below to instantly access your downloadable book.

***

Bonus #3 – Life Skills for Teens and Young Adults

Unlock real-world tools to build independence, confidence, and success!

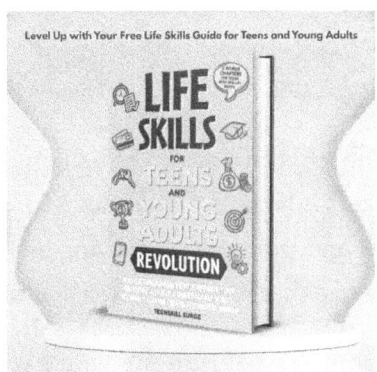

Ready to dive deeper?
Scan the QR code to download your free companion book and continue your journey!

Introduction

Y ou're standing in the school hallway. The bell rings, people hurry past, and a group by the lockers is laughing. You spot a friend in the crowd, but she doesn't look up. For a second, you consider saying hi—then that familiar ache settles in your chest, the one that whispers, *"You don't belong here."*

Later, while scrolling through your phone, you see a weekend selfie with faces you know—everyone except yours. Suddenly, you feel smaller, like you're fading into the background. Maybe you've asked yourself, *"What's wrong with me? Why does it always seem like everyone else has it together?"*

If any of this rings true, you're in the right place. I wrote this handbook to remind you that even when life feels loud, confusing, or lonely, you still belong. You're not broken, you're not behind, and you're definitely not the only one who feels this way.

I'm Monika. For years, I've listened to girls talk about the pressure, self-doubt, and constant stress that come with growing up in a world that never seems to slow down. I wrote this book because I know what it's like to feel left out, to lie awake worrying, and to wonder whether you'll ever feel "enough." I know how easy it is to scroll through perfect pictures and wonder why everyone else seems happier or more confident. No one deserves to feel invisible or like they have to change who they are just to be accepted.

I hope that this book helps you feel seen, valued, and grounded—not just for a moment, but in how you see yourself every day. I want to give you tools that actually make life lighter—things you can *do*, not just think about. No sugar-coated advice, no tired "just be yourself" lines. You deserve real answers that fit your world.

Let's be honest: being a teen today is hard. Maybe your group chat blows up with inside jokes you're not part of. Maybe school feels like a mountain you can't climb. Perhaps you look in the mirror and see a version of yourself that doesn't feel "enough." The truth is, so many girls feel exactly like this, even the ones who seem like they have it all together. Your feelings are real. They matter. And you are not alone.

This book isn't a lecture or a list of rules. Think of it as a big sister who gets it—someone who's walked through the awkward, messy stuff and made it out stronger (and maybe even laughed about it later). I'm sharing what I've learned from research, from talking with real girls, and from my own imperfect life. We'll speak honestly, laugh when we can, and sit with the hard stuff when we have to—no judgment, no fake positivity, and absolutely no "get over it" nonsense.

Inside, you'll find honest answers and simple, realistic steps for the things you face every day:

Friendships that sometimes feel like rollercoasters — how to spot real friends, set boundaries, and handle conflict without losing yourself.

Social media that messes with your confidence — how to enjoy it without letting likes decide your worth.

School pressure that feels endless — how to calm your nerves, manage your time, and take small breaks without guilt.

Body image and self-worth — how to see your reflection with kindness, not comparison.

We'll keep things real—no pressure to be perfect, no one-size-fits-all solutions. Just tools, stories, and reflections that help you handle life with a little more confidence and a lot more self-compassion.

You don't have to have everything figured out to start feeling better. You need small steps that make sense for *you*.

Above all, I want you to remember this: you don't have to shrink to fit anyone else's idea of who you should be. You are already enough—messy, quiet, bold, scared, intense, imperfect, and absolutely worthy.

So take a deep breath. Exhale slowly. You're here now. This is your space to grow, laugh, and rediscover what makes you, *you*. Turn the page when you're ready—we'll figure it out together. You've got this. And I've got your back.

Chapter 1

You're Not Alone

The Real Truth About Feeling Left Out

Some moments stick with you—a loud cafeteria, a group laughing together. At the same time, you hover at the edge, unsure if there's room for you. Maybe you look for a friendly wave and end up scrolling through your phone, pretending you're busy so no one notices you're alone. That ache in your chest is real. Questions start to pile up: *Did I say something wrong? Am I too quiet? Too much? Why does it seem like everyone else has a place except me?*

It can feel like everyone else holds a secret you somehow missed. But here's the truth: feeling left out is one of the most common experiences in the world. Almost everyone you see—even those with big friend groups or confident vibes—has felt invisible at some point. Exclusion isn't a sign that something's wrong with you. It's something almost everyone goes through at some point in life.

***

WHY EVERYONE FEELS LEFT OUT (EVEN THE "POPULAR" GIRLS)

Let's clear something up: feeling excluded doesn't only happen to shy or quiet girls. It can happen to anyone—athletes, performers, top students, or those with thousands of followers. People are really good at hiding loneliness behind smiles and highlight reels.

Take **Jamie**, a sophomore who made varsity soccer as a first-year student. She seemed to have it all—friends, confidence, recognition. But she once told me she cried after finding a group chat where her name was missing. "My name wasn't even in the conversation," she said quietly. That kind of sting hits harder than people realize.

Social media makes it worse. You scroll through perfect photos, seeing classmates at parties, laughing in stories that look effortless and fun. What you don't see is what's missing from the frame. A girl known for her TikTok dances might look like friends surround her, but she told me she spent an entire weekend alone while her "close friends" went on a trip without her. *"People assume I'm never lonely,"* she said, *"but that weekend I watched their stories and pretended it didn't bother me."*

Followers aren't the same as friends. Being seen online doesn't mean being known in real life.

Even girls who seem "in" the group sometimes feel like outsiders. One student told me, *"I'm part of the group, but I always feel like the backup friend—like I'm there because they need an extra person."* Another said, *"I'm always the one taking the pictures, not in them."* These moments sound small, but they build up, leaving you wondering if you'll ever truly belong.

Popularity, followers, or a packed calendar don't protect anyone from feeling left out. Theater kids, gamers, musicians, artists—everyone has their own version of exclusion. Sometimes you're left out of a party. Other times, you're left out of a conversation, a group text, or even a joke that everyone else gets. What you see on the outside rarely matches what's happening inside someone else's head.

Social media makes that gap even wider. We see highlight reels—perfect smiles, surprise parties, big friend groups—without the arguments, awkward silences, or tears that came before or after. If you compared Instagram stories to real life, you'd see how much gets edited away—by filters, by captions, by what people choose to show.

Here's something most people won't say out loud: **being surrounded by people who don't honestly know you can feel lonelier than being alone.** Sometimes the person in the middle of the crowd feels more invisible than the one sitting by herself.

***

What Feeling Left Out Teaches You

It hurts, yes—but it's not meaningless. Feeling left out shows you how deeply you care about belonging and connection. It means your heart notices what matters. Sometimes, moments like these help you find where you *don't* belong—so you can make space for people and places that make you feel safe and accepted.

When you start noticing that nearly everyone has felt this ache, it loses some of its power. It's not just your story—it's part of being human. And it doesn't define your worth.

Remember this: you can't always control who includes you, but you can control how you care for yourself in those moments. You can reach out to one kind person instead of trying to impress a whole group. You can remind yourself that belonging isn't about fitting in everywhere—it's about finding where you're valued for who you are.

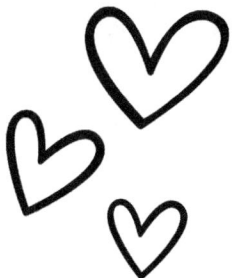

Journaling Prompt

- Take a few minutes and write about a time you felt left out.

- Start with the *scene*: Where were you? Who was there? What was happening?

- Then, go deeper—what did it feel like inside your body? Did your chest tighten? Did your stomach drop? What thoughts ran through your mind? Be completely honest—no censoring or editing.

Next, ask yourself:

- What do I wish people understood about me in that moment?

- What kind of connection was I really craving?

- What might I say now to comfort the version of me in that memory?

You'll probably notice something powerful: almost everyone has felt this way. Naming it helps you release it. It makes it easier to talk about what you need, to reach out, and to remind yourself that being left out isn't the same as being unworthy.

***

A Little Truth to Take With You

Everyone has invisible moments—times when they wonder if they're enough or if anyone sees them. But connection starts with honesty, not perfection. When you allow yourself to be real—awkward, silly, emotional—you make space for others to be real too. That's how belonging begins.

You are not behind. You're not broken. You're simply learning how to find people who make room for the real you. And that's one of the bravest things you'll ever do.

***

DECODING SOCIAL CIRCLES — WHY GROUPS FORM AND SHIFT

Friend groups at school can feel like living things—constantly growing, shrinking, or rearranging themselves in ways that don't always make sense. One week, everything feels solid; the next, you're staring at an empty seat at lunch or noticing a new group laughing by the vending machines.

It's easy to assume that means something's wrong with you—but most of the time, it's not personal. Friend circles change because people change. And understanding *why* it happens can help you stop blaming yourself when the people around you start shifting.

***

Why Groups Form (and Why They Shift So Much)

There's an invisible pattern behind most friend groups. People naturally form circles around things that make them feel safe or understood. Psychologists call this the *in-group/out-group* effect—but you've probably seen it in real life without even realizing it.

You might notice how the art kids sit together, the basketball team huddles over lunch, or the choir crew takes over a corner of the hallway before rehearsal. It's not because anyone planned it that way—it just happens. We all gravitate toward people who "get" us.

But here's the catch: those circles aren't permanent. They expand and contract with every new semester, team, or class project. One small change—a new club, a schedule switch, or even a new seating chart—can shift the entire social landscape.

It's not a sign you've done something wrong. It's just part of growing up and discovering who fits into your world right now.

***

When Change Feels Personal (But Isn't)

Transitions accelerate friendship changes. Moving schools, joining a club, switching sports teams—each one reshuffles who you spend the most time with.

Someone who used to sit with childhood friends might suddenly find herself spending every afternoon at rehearsal with the theater crew. Another might trade weekend hangouts for late-night study sessions with a new lab partner.

That doesn't mean the old friendships don't matter. Sometimes life builds new bridges faster than we can cross them.

Still, it can hurt to see an old group grow closer without you. It's natural to feel left out or even guilty—like you're betraying your past friendships. But the truth is, **drifting doesn't always mean losing.** Sometimes it's just making space for new connections that fit the version of you that's growing.

***

THE UNSPOKEN RULES INSIDE FRIEND GROUPS

Every friend group has its own rhythm—shared playlists, inside jokes, memes, and the unwritten rule of who plans hangouts. Usually, the person who spends the most time with others ends up organizing things, so the invites often go to whoever's closest at the moment.

So when you're left out of a group chat or not invited to a movie night, it doesn't always mean someone purposely excluded you. Sometimes it's just timing. People fall into patterns: a quick conversation turns into a plan, and before anyone notices, the group looks slightly different from the way it did last week.

It's frustrating, yes—but it's rarely as intentional as it feels.

***

Drifting vs. Being Excluded

There's a difference between *drifting* and *being excluded.*

Drifting happens quietly. Schedules get busy, interests shift, and texts slow down.

Exclusion feels sharper—like being talked about, ignored, or blocked online.

Most social changes fall into the *drifting* category. That doesn't mean it doesn't hurt, but it does change what you can do about it. Drifting invites reflection and curiosity; exclusion might require boundaries and new connections.

Understanding which one you're experiencing helps you choose your next step with clarity instead of panic.

Mapping Your Circle

Watching your social world with curiosity (not self-blame) teaches you a lot about patterns of connection. Try this quick visual activity—it's not about judging anyone, just noticing dynamics:

> **Draw your friend's map.** Put yourself in the middle. Add circles for each friend or group.
> **Connect lines.** Who hangs out most often? Who plans things? Who floats between groups?
> **Notice your role.** Are you the organizer? The listener? The go-between?
> **Reflect.** Are these relationships balanced, or do they feel one-sided?

Once you see the map, ask: *What feels healthy here—and what doesn't?*

This awareness gives you power. It's not about forcing people to include you; it's about deciding where your energy belongs.

You can:

Keep showing up for the people who care.

Create your own hangouts and see who joins.

Or gently step back from connections that no longer feel mutual.

***

Stories That Make Sense of It All

Lila, a ninth-grader, thought her middle school besties were her "forever people." But when she joined the art club, her after-school hours shifted. Paint-stained fingers and shared canvases built new bonds, and sleepovers turned into sketch nights. At first, she felt guilty. Then she realized she could hold space for both—her old friends and her new ones.

Zoe had the opposite experience. Her group stopped inviting her after she quit volleyball. She spent a few lonely months trying to figure out what she'd done wrong—until a class project paired her with someone quiet but kind. Study sessions turned into inside jokes and spontaneous coffee runs. That friendship didn't look flashy, but it felt real—and it lasted.

Every story has a turning point. Most friendship shifts aren't about fault; they're about growth.

Reflection Prompt
- Grab your journal and think about this:

- What friendship patterns do you notice around you?

- Is there a group or person you've been holding onto even though it no longer feels right?

- What kind of friendships make you feel calm, safe, and accepted?

Write freely. Be honest with yourself. Sometimes letting go of what's shifting gives you space to discover where you truly belong.

***

The Takeaway

Friendships change shape as you change. That's not rejection—it's realignment.

Groups grow, fade, and reform. People come and go. But your worth stays constant.

When you understand *why* circles shift, you stop trying to chase belonging—and start creating it.

***

FOMO IRL: When You See Friends Hanging Out Without You

Nothing stings quite like unlocking your phone and seeing a group selfie from Friday night—a sleepover you didn't even know was happening. Everyone's laughing, their arms wrapped around each other, faces glowing in fairy-light filters. The caption is full of emojis and inside jokes you don't get, while your notifications stay quiet.

Sometimes the ache shows up in real life, too. You walk past the lunch table and hear that familiar laugh—the one you know by heart—but this time it isn't shared with you. You slow your steps, hoping for a wave or a glance, but it never comes. It feels like being a ghost in a room full of voices.

That sinking feeling in your chest? That's FOMO—*fear of missing out.* But it's more than just jealousy. It's that deep, hollow ache of feeling unseen, like you're standing outside a window watching the world move without you. Your heart beats a little faster—your stomach knots. Thoughts start to swirl: *Did they forget me? Did I do something wrong? Am I not fun enough anymore?*

When that ache hits, it's easy to believe the story your brain tells first—the one that says, *You don't matter*. But there's always more to the story than what you see on your screen.

***

Why It Hurts So Much

Social media magnifies everything. One picture, one tag, one caption—suddenly it feels like proof that you were left out on purpose. Screenshots of group chats, "wish you were here!" posts, and endless highlight reels can make your world shrink to a pinpoint of "not invited."

What you don't see are the missing pieces. You don't see the awkward silences between photos, the friend who didn't actually want to be there, or the group text that started five minutes before the invite went out. Social media doesn't tell you the whole story—it just zooms in on the happiest moment and cuts out the rest.

Everyone, even the people who seem perfectly confident, has had that moment of wondering why they were omitted. You're not the only one staring at your phone, feeling that wave of emptiness. You're not the only one who's cried quietly because something you cared about happened without you. You're not alone in this.

***

When Your Mind Starts to Spiral

FOMO is sneaky. It doesn't just hurt—it pulls you into a loop of comparison and overthinking. That's when you can try something small but mighty: pause.

Set your phone down, even for a minute. Take a slow, deliberate breath. Notice where you are—the pattern on your bedsheet, the hum of the refrigerator, the sound of your own breathing. Name three things you can see right now. Listen for one sound nearby.

This isn't about pretending you're not sad. It's about reminding your body that you're safe in this moment. When your thoughts start racing toward *why not me?*, your body can gently answer, *"I'm okay right now."* Sometimes, calm starts one breath at a time.

***

Untangling the Story in Your Head

When you're hurt, your mind fills in the blanks with the harshest possibilities. You might catch yourself thinking, *They didn't want me there*, or *I'm not important enough to invite.*

But here's the truth: feelings are real, but thoughts aren't always facts.

Try to notice what story you're telling yourself about what happened. Then ask: *Could there be another explanation?*

It could be a last-minute plan. Space was limited. Maybe they assumed you were busy or just forgot to hit send. The point isn't to excuse anyone—it's to give your brain more than one path to travel. When you believe only the worst story, it hurts twice as much.

Changing your inner story takes practice. It can feel strange at first, but it's an act of kindness toward yourself. Try whispering things like, *This hurts, but it doesn't mean I'm unworthy.* Or, *people sometimes forget, but I still matter.*

These phrases aren't magic spells, but they soften the edges of pain. They make space for self-compassion to step in where shame once lived. Be kind to yourself in these moments.

***

Choosing What Comes Next

Once the sharpness fades a little, ask yourself: *What do I want to do now?*

You don't have to pretend it didn't hurt, and you don't have to lash out either. Sometimes the healthiest thing is to reach out—not to accuse, but to reconnect. You might text something simple, like, *"Hey, I saw the pics—it looked fun! Would love to join next time."* Or, *"Miss hanging out—want to grab coffee this weekend?"*

People can be thoughtless, but not always intentionally hurtful. Most of the time, no one realizes someone was left out until it's already happened. Speaking up is brave. It reminds others you still want to be included—and it reminds *you* that your voice matters.

If texting feels like too much, shift the focus back to yourself. Do something that helps you feel alive again. Go for a walk with music that makes you feel strong. Make pancakes just for you. Paint your nails, journal in color, dance in your room, play a game, organize your desk.

These little moments aren't distractions—they're declarations. They say, *My joy belongs to me, not to a group chat.*

***

When the Sadness Stays

Sometimes, even after you've done all the right things—breathed, written, walked—the sadness sticks around. That's okay. It doesn't mean you're broken or weak. It means you have a heart that notices connection and misses it when it's gone.

Try talking to someone who understands. Maybe an older sibling, a cousin, or a friend who's had a similar moment. Sometimes saying the words out loud releases their power. You might even laugh together about how dramatic FOMO can make us all feel.

And when you're alone, try this gentle reminder: *It's okay to feel hurt. I still matter.*

Repeat it if you need to. Out loud. Whisper it like a secret promise. You are worthy of love and inclusion. You matter.

Being left out doesn't erase your value. It only means that in this moment, your story is taking a different turn—and that story is still worth showing up for.

Journaling Moment

If you're ready to unpack the feelings, try writing about what triggered your FOMO. What did you see, hear, or imagine? Then finish these sentences in your notebook:

"The story I'm telling myself is..."

"Another possible explanation could be..."

When you're done, notice what it feels like to hold both ideas at once. Most of the time, the truth sits somewhere between them.

Before you close your journal, add one more line: *"Tonight, I'll do something kind for myself because I still matter."* Then follow through, even in a small way.

Missing out hurts, and that pain is real. But it doesn't mean you're unworthy of joy, friendship, or belonging. The world hasn't forgotten you; it's just still in motion, and your part of the story isn't done yet.

Even when it feels like everyone else is being chosen first, remember: your story isn't happening in someone else's post. It's unfolding right here, in the quiet courage it takes to keep showing up.

You belong, with or without a tag.

***

Turning Awkward Moments Into Connection Opportunities

Awkwardness has a way of making you feel like the only person in the room who doesn't know what to do with their hands. It can feel like a bright spotlight you never asked for—your cheeks burn, your stomach twists, and you silently wish for a trapdoor to open beneath you.

But here's the truth: everyone, *absolutely everyone*, has awkward moments. Even the people who look perfectly confident on the outside have said something weird, tripped at the worst possible time, or waved to someone who wasn't actually waving at them. Awkwardness doesn't mean something's wrong with you—it's proof you're human, and that everyone else is, too.

Picture this: you're hurrying through the hallway, arms full of books, and suddenly one slips, then another. The clatter echoes, your face flushes, and you're sure everyone saw. Most people freeze in those moments, hoping invisibility is absolute. But sometimes, someone nearby laughs—not cruelly, but kindly—and starts helping you gather the mess. For a second, the embarrassment fades and turns into something warmer: a shared moment of realness.

Awkwardness isn't a flaw to erase. It's a bridge waiting to be crossed.

***

THE HIDDEN GIFT OF AWKWARDNESS

A lot of friendships don't start with movie-perfect introductions. They begin in small, messy moments—a shared cringe, a wrong word, or a laugh that comes out too loud. Awkwardness connects people because it strips away the pretending.

When you start to see these moments not as disasters but as *openings*, something shifts. The silence in class that makes you want to disappear? You could turn to the person next to you and whisper, *"I never know what to say when it gets this quiet."* If your stomach growls mid-test and someone laughs, you could grin and say, *"Guess I should've eaten that granola bar."* These small comments turn tension into connection.

The goal isn't to be smooth—it's to be real. Because people don't remember flawless conversations, they remember genuine ones.

***

Owning the Moment

You don't need a perfect line ready for every awkward situation. What matters most is *owning the moment* instead of running from it.

If you meet someone new and stumble over your words, you can smile and say, *"That came out weird—let me try again."* When you spill your drink, laugh instead of apologizing fifty times. A little humor softens the moment for everyone, including you.

Confidence isn't about never feeling awkward. It's about being okay with it when it happens. The more you practice owning your quirks, the lighter awkwardness becomes.

Kindness Starts with Noticing

Some of the best connections happen when you notice someone else's awkwardness and respond with kindness. There may be a classmate who lingers at the edge of your group, pretending to scroll their phone while everyone else talks. Or the new student who hovers near the lunch line, unsure where to sit.

Those moments are invitations. The tiniest gesture—a smile, a *"hey,"* or a simple *"want to sit here?"*—can change someone's whole day.

If you start paying attention, you'll see quiet signs all around you: someone looking down when laughter starts, someone's eyes darting around a crowded room, someone nodding but not really joining in. You don't need to analyze anyone, just be aware. Empathy grows when you see what others might be feeling, even if they never say it out loud.

And when you're brave enough to make that first move—to invite someone in—you also start healing the parts of you that have ever felt left out.

A Small Challenge

This week, choose one moment to reach out.

It doesn't have to be huge—invite someone to join your table, include a classmate in your group project, or walk with someone new between classes.

Even if they say no, your effort still matters. You'll never know how much your small act of kindness could mean to someone who needed it. Sometimes being seen once is enough to remind someone they belong.

And if the thought of reaching out feels terrifying, start with something tiny—eye contact, a genuine smile, or a *"Hey, how's it going?"* Small steps count.

***

Awkward Doesn't Mean Broken

The thing about awkward moments is that they shrink with time. What feels like the end of the world today often becomes a story you laugh about later.

Think about a time you were embarrassed—a tripped step, a stuttered hello, a moment your joke flopped and landed flat. If you look back, chances are it wasn't as catastrophic as it felt. In fact, those moments often become the glue that holds new friendships together.

One reader told me about her "disaster" science presentation, where she mispronounced *mitochondria* and froze mid-sentence. She admitted it out loud—*"I have no idea what I'm saying right now"*—and braced for laughter. But her partner just smiled and said, *"Same here."* That small bit of honesty turned into a study partnership and, eventually, a real friendship.

Another girl told me she once spilled her smoothie across the lunch table on her first day at a new school. Instead of running away, she stayed to clean up, apologizing through tears. Two classmates helped her, joked about the "sticky start," and the three of them ended up inseparable by spring.

These stories aren't rare—they're reminders that awkwardness doesn't end connection; it begins it.

***

Reflecting on Your Own Moments

If there's an awkward memory that still pops into your mind and makes you cringe, it might help to explore it instead of avoiding it.

Write about what happened—what you said, how you felt, what you noticed afterward. Then ask yourself: Did anyone actually judge me, or did I imagine they did? Did something good come out of it later, even a small laugh or moment of understanding?

If you could go back and talk to your past self in that moment, what would you say? Maybe you'd say, *"You're okay,"* or, *"You're still worthy even when you blush."*

You'll probably realize that no single awkward moment defines you—and that you survived all of them.

***

Closing Reflection

Every awkward stumble, every pause, every too-loud laugh carries a tiny thread of connection waiting to be noticed.

When you stop treating awkwardness like a problem to hide and start seeing it as proof that you're alive, it loses its power to isolate you.

Sometimes, the most memorable friendships begin in the cracks—between spilled drinks and nervous hellos, in the honesty of "me too."

You don't have to perfect your words or timing to be loved. You have to keep showing up, imperfect and real, because that's the version of you the world needs most.

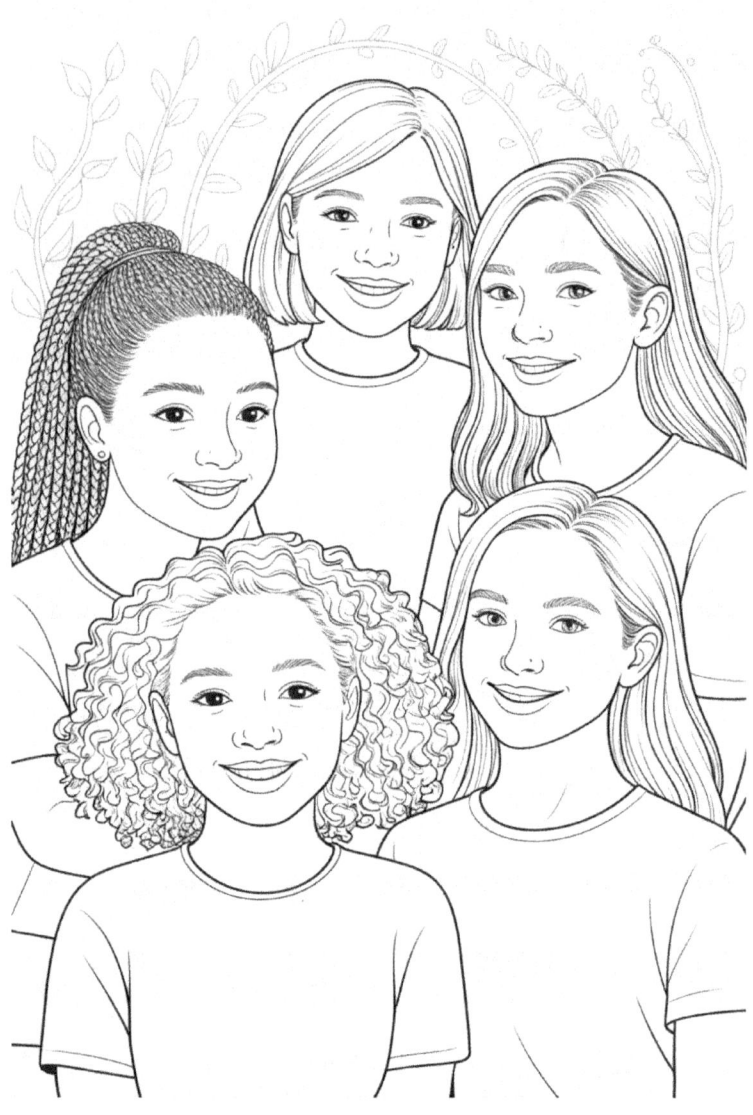

Chapter 2

Friendship Drama

Navigating the Hard Stuff Without Losing Yourself

Friendship is supposed to feel safe—like slipping into your favorite hoodie or replaying a song that always hits right. Yet sometimes something that once felt light starts to feel heavy. Maybe every hangout turns into a therapy session for your friend's problems, or you leave feeling drained instead of happy. You can't quite name it, but something feels off.

That discomfort doesn't make you "too sensitive." It means your instincts are trying to protect you.

Healthy friendships should add peace, not pressure. They feel balanced—you can be yourself, disagree without fear, and know your laughter or silence won't be used against you later. After spending time together, you feel lighter, not smaller. Kindness moves both ways: your secrets stay private, your boundaries matter, and your wins are celebrated instead of minimized. In a healthy friendship, no one keeps score or guilt-trips you for having other friends. There's space for honesty and for apologies when things go wrong.

But sometimes the balance shifts. What starts as teasing becomes humiliation. The person who used to hype you up now criticizes your clothes or jokes about you in front of others. Maybe they control who you talk to, demand constant attention, or go silent when you say no. They might also spread rumors, pressure you into choices that feel wrong, or call you "too sensitive" when you try to speak up.

Toxic behavior often begins quietly and grows louder over time—until you start to doubt yourself. When you identify these signs, it's not a reflection of your sensitivity, but rather a testament to your self-awareness and strength. Trusting your instincts is a powerful tool in protecting yourself from toxic relationships.

***

FRIENDSHIP GREEN AND RED FLAGS (WHAT THEY REALLY MEAN)

Think of these not as a checklist to memorize but as snapshots of how a friendship might sound or feel.

When it's healthy, conversations flow both ways. Your friend listens, asks questions, and respects your boundaries. They show up when life gets messy, not just when it's convenient. They can laugh at mistakes without turning them into weapons. You both feel safe to say *"I'm sorry"* or *"I need space."*

When it's unhealthy, the pattern flips. Maybe they interrupt or ignore what you say, show up only when they need something, or guilt-trip you for spending time elsewhere. They might tease you about things that really hurt, or break your confidence by sharing private details you trusted them with. Instead of resolving conflict, they might explode with anger or freeze you out until you apologize for something you didn't do.

If this sounds familiar, it's not drama—it's imbalance.

***

The Confusion That Follows

Questioning a friendship can feel like standing on shaky ground. Part of you notices the tension; another part whispers, But we've known each other forever. Loyalty runs deep, especially if that friend once made you feel special. You may tell yourself it's just a rough patch or that everyone fights sometimes. And yes, no friendship is perfect. But real friends don't make your stomach drop when their name pops up on your screen.

It's normal to feel torn between guilt and exhaustion. Walking away can seem scarier than staying, because at least staying is familiar. Yet staying in something that hurts doesn't make you loyal—it makes you invisible to yourself.

***

Empower Yourself by tuning in to Your Own Signals

Before every hangout, pause and notice how you feel. Are you excited or uneasy? While you're together, do you feel relaxed or careful with every word? Afterward, do you replay conversations, worrying that you said the wrong thing?

Those small gut feelings are your truth quietly showing up, bringing a sense of relief. Over time, patterns reveal what your heart already knows. If you've felt dismissed, pressured, or drained more than once, your body is sending data your brain can trust.

Being self-aware is crucial in maintaining healthy relationships. A healthy friendship leaves you recharged. A toxic one leaves you second-guessing everything.

A Moment of Reflection

Take a moment to reflect on your friendship. Grab a notebook and answer this:

- How do I feel before, during, and after time with this friend?

- Write down a few memories—times you felt ignored, uncomfortable, or guilty for saying no. What happened, and how did you react? Did you talk to anyone about it? Seeing the words in front of you helps separate emotion from pattern.

You might realize the problem isn't one bad day; it's a recurring ache that deserves attention.

***

Stories from the Real World

One reader shared how her "best friend" always vanished when life got hard. During exams and stress, she'd be alone, but once things calmed down, the friend reappeared with new gossip as if nothing had happened. She finally noticed the pattern: support flowed only one way.

Another girl described a friend who constantly crossed boundaries—borrowing clothes without asking, reading messages over her shoulder, brushing off requests for privacy as *"you're so dramatic."* After months of confusion and guilt, she decided to step back. At first, she felt lonely; then she felt free. *"I can finally breathe again,"* she said.

These stories are a reminder that prioritizing your well-being is not a betrayal, but an act of self-respect.

***

Why Leaving Hurts Even When It's Right

Ending a friendship, especially one woven into your everyday life, can feel like ripping a chapter out of your own story. You lose shared jokes, routines, and someone who once felt like home. That grief is real. But the peace that follows—a quiet that doesn't carry tension—is the space where healing begins.

You deserve friendships that celebrate your growth, not fear it. You deserve to walk away from conversations feeling heard, not hollow.

***

Learning to Trust Yourself Again

Toxic dynamics often teach you to doubt your own perspective. You start asking, Am I overreacting? Maybe I'm the problem. It takes time to rebuild trust in yourself. Start small. Notice the moments when your body tightens or your mood drops. Believe that information.

Then remember: healthy love—whether from a friend, partner, or family member—never requires you to shrink.

The more you practice listening inward, the easier it becomes to protect your energy without apology.

***

If You're Not Ready to Walk Away Yet

Sometimes the friendship isn't all bad. There are still good memories, reasons to hope it could improve. If that's where you are, you can start by setting small boundaries instead of cutting ties overnight.

Try saying, *"I can't talk right now, but let's catch up later,"* or *"I don't feel comfortable with that."* A real friend will pause, adjust, and care about how their choices affect you. If they roll their eyes, guilt-trip you, or twist your words—that reaction is its own answer.

Change begins when you stop explaining why you deserve respect.

A Short Reflection Exercise

Close your eyes for a moment and picture a friendship that feels peaceful.

What does it look like? How do you act when you're with them?

Now, picture the one that drains you. What shifts inside you—your posture, your breathing, your tone?

That contrast tells you everything you need to know.

Write one promise to yourself: *I will protect the friendships that help me grow, and release the ones that make me doubt who I am.*

***

Moving Forward

Friendship drama hurts because it cuts close to identity—it's about who sees you and who doesn't. But each red flag you notice and act on strengthens your confidence. Every time you choose calm over chaos, you reclaim a little more of your energy.

It's OK to miss the person and still know they're not right for you anymore. It's OK to feel sad and still sure.

Leaving space in your life doesn't create emptiness; it creates room for people who meet you with honesty, laughter, and care—the kind of friends who don't make your stomach drop when they text, who celebrate your quirks instead of using them as punchlines.

That's the friendship you deserve.

***

When Friends Turn Cold — Navigating Exclusion with Strength and Grace

Suddenly finding yourself outside a friend group you once called your second family can shake you to your core. The silence in the group chat feels louder than a slammed door. Maybe it started with something small—a misunderstanding that never got cleared up—or perhaps you just thought it: the replies grew shorter, the invites slowed down, and the inside jokes multiplied without you.

It's not only the loneliness that hurts. It's the confusion. You replay conversations in your head, searching for what you said wrong. You scroll through old photos, wondering when things changed. One girl put it perfectly: *"It's like I became invisible overnight."*

That numb, lost feeling can make you question everything—even your worth.

***

It's Not Always About You

Your brain will immediately try to make sense of what happened by blaming you. But friendship shifts happen for so many reasons that have nothing to do with your value. Sometimes people grow in different directions. Sometimes someone is dealing with something private. Sometimes drama spreads faster than the truth ever could.

Even knowing that doesn't make it hurt less. The ache shows up in small ways — passing your old table in the cafeteria, hearing your favorite song play in the background of their new video, or seeing their weekend photos pop up while you're home alone. You might hold your breath every time you check your phone, hoping for a message that never comes. The question *why me?* Echoes so loud it drowns out everything else.

But here's what's true: your worth doesn't disappear just because someone stopped seeing it.

***

When You're Ready to Reach Out

When friends go distant, it takes courage to reach out instead of shutting down. You might fear being ignored or, worse, rejected. Still, honest communication—spoken calmly, without blame—can sometimes clear the air or at least give you closure.

If you decide to reach out, keep it simple and kind. You could say something like:

"Hey, I've noticed we haven't talked much lately. Is everything OK between us?"

"If I did something to upset you, I'd really like to talk about it."

"I miss hanging out. Are we OK?"

These small words open a big door. You're not begging for attention—you're showing maturity, courage, and care for yourself. Whether they respond or not, you've chosen honesty over silence, and that's powerful.

***

When the Silence Stays

Sometimes reaching out won't change the outcome. The replies might stay short or never come at all. That sting cuts deep, but it's also a turning point—a moment to choose your own peace.

When others grow cold, don't let their silence freeze your sense of worth. Try whispering to yourself: *I am worthy of genuine friendship, even if this group can't see it.* Write it on a note. Make it your lock screen. Say it out loud in the mirror if you need to. This simple act of kindness toward yourself matters more than you think.

The goal isn't to convince anyone to stay. It's to remind yourself that you still belong somewhere—even if it's not here anymore.

***

Finding Warmth Elsewhere

While you're healing, lean on your "support squad"—the people who genuinely care. That could be a sibling who always makes you laugh, a cousin who texts you memes, a teacher who listens, a coach who believes in you, or even an online friend who's seen your heart through a screen.

Sometimes one honest, quiet conversation can heal more than a hundred unread messages. Let the people who make you feel safe know you could use some company. They don't have to fix it—they have to listen.

And if talking feels too raw right now, express what you're feeling another way.

Draw. Write. Bake. Sing. Run. Create. Do something that reminds you there's more to you than this moment of exclusion. Healing doesn't always happen through words; sometimes it happens through motion, through art, through life continuing in your hands.

***

Learning from What Happened

Reflecting on what happened isn't about assigning blame—it's about learning who you are and what kind of energy you want around you.

Ask yourself: *What truly matters to me in a friend?*

It could be someone who checks in when things are hard, who keeps your secrets safe, who celebrates your wins without turning them into competition. Perhaps it's someone who makes space for your boundaries, not someone who pushes past them.

You might even write out a list—not as homework, but as a reminder of what a healthy connection looks like in your life.

For example, you might say:

"A good friend listens without judging."

"They remember the small things that matter to me."

"They support me when I mess up."

"They make time even when life's busy."

"They respect my values and boundaries."

"They laugh with me—not at me."

"They admit when they're wrong and try to make it right."

Every line you write is a reflection of the kind of love you deserve—and the kind you'll start to attract when you believe in it.

Journaling Moment

After a cold patch or fallout, find a quiet space and write about what you've learned. Start with this line:

"What did I learn from this experience?"

Let your words flow, even if they're messy, angry, or sad. You may realize you're stronger than you thought. You may see patterns in how you give more than you receive. Or you'll discover what kind of friend you want to be next time.

This isn't about moving on—it's about moving forward with more clarity and more self-respect.

***

Opening Up to New Circles

Even when one group fades away, the connection isn't over. New friendships can grow where you least expect them—sitting next to someone new in class, chatting with a neighbor, or joining a club or volunteer group. Sometimes the right people are already in your orbit, quietly waiting for space to open.

Keep showing up as yourself—your curious, funny, imperfect, amazing self. The right friends will recognize you not for how perfectly you fit in, but for how real you are.

One day, you'll look back at this moment and realize it wasn't an ending at all. It was the beginning of something more genuine—something built on mutual care, not convenience.

You don't have to shrink to fit someone else's circle. The people meant for you will create space for you to stand tall.

***

A Closing Thought

Losing friends can feel like losing pieces of yourself. But sometimes, those spaces are where new growth begins.

You are not defined by who leaves you out.

You are defined by how you choose to keep your heart open anyway.

Keep showing up—with kindness, with courage, and with faith that the right people will meet you where you are because they will.

***

RUMORS, GROUP CHATS, AND SNAP STREAKS: HANDLING DIGITAL DRAMA

Digital drama can sting deeper than real-life fights. Sometimes it starts with a single notification—a tag, a post, a "joke" that doesn't land—and suddenly your name is everywhere. Comments pile up. Screenshots spread faster than you can breathe. And before you know it, you've become the topic of a conversation you never agreed to join.

You might open your phone and find your group chat sitting at the center of it all. A message meant as sarcasm is shared outside the chat and suddenly comes across as cruel. Inside jokes turn into something sharp. The words twist, context disappears, and suddenly it feels like everyone's looking at you differently.

Online, things escalate in seconds. The people piling on aren't always trying to be cruel—sometimes they don't even realize how far it's gone. But for the person on the receiving end, it can feel like being surrounded by noise you can't silence.

***

Before You React

The urge to fire back is strong. You want to defend yourself, to correct the story, to make the noise stop. But that first impulse—the angry reply, the *"let me explain"*—often feeds the fire instead of putting it out.

Before you respond, pause. Put your phone down for a few minutes. Breathe deeply, even if it feels pointless. Give yourself time to think before your thumbs start typing.

When you're ready, gather the facts. Screenshot anything cruel, threatening, or harassing. Not because you're being dramatic—but because having evidence protects you if things need to be reported later.

Then mute the notifications. Seriously. You're allowed to take back control of your headspace. You don't need every buzz and ping pulling you back into pain.

After that, talk it through with someone outside the drama—a parent, teacher, sibling, or friend who isn't involved. Telling the story out loud often makes it less tangled in your mind. Someone you trust can help you see the situation with clearer eyes.

***

If You Choose to Respond

Sometimes you'll decide it's worth speaking up—especially if a rumor or lie is spreading. In that case, keep your message calm, short, and direct. Something like:

"Hey, I saw what's being said. That's not true, and it's hurtful to see it going around."

That's enough. You don't owe anyone a long explanation. State the truth, then step back.

If people keep pushing, remember that silence is also a response. You can leave the chat, stop replying, or block anyone who's trying to stir things up. Protecting your peace isn't weakness—**it's wisdom**. It's a courageous and wise choice that can empower and make you feel confident.

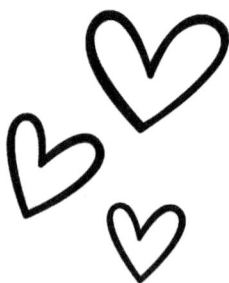

Pause Before You Post

Whenever you feel pulled into digital drama, ask yourself:

- Have I taken a breath before replying?

- Would I say this to their face?

- Is what I'm about to post respectful?

- Am I sharing facts or just feelings?

- Do I even need to respond at all?

Nine times out of ten, waiting even a few minutes changes what you want to say—and how you want to say it. Sometimes the most potent response is none at all.

One girl told me she wrote a long, angry paragraph in Notes but never sent it. She just needed to release it safely. Later, she said, "Not posting it was the best thing I ever did for my sanity."

***

Creating Digital Boundaries

Muting or leaving group chats, blocking accounts, and taking breaks from apps are not overreactions—they're survival skills. You are not obligated to stay connected to anyone or anything that drains your peace. It's a powerful act of self-care that can bring relief and empowerment if someone calls you dramatic for needing space; that says more about them than it ever will about you.

Snapchat streaks, for example, can feel like friendship scorecards. Breaking one can feel like betrayal—but your worth isn't measured in fire emojis. Sometimes letting a streak end is the healthiest thing you can do.

One reader shared that after a minor misunderstanding blew up in her group, her Snap notifications turned into nonstop pings. Every buzz made her stomach drop. She finally muted the app for a week. She worried she'd lose friends, but something surprising happened: the people who really cared reached out offline. Her anxiety dropped. Her friendships—at least the real ones—remained.

Taking space online doesn't mean you're disappearing. It means you're choosing to breathe.

***

How to Step Back Gracefully

If you want to exit a toxic chat without stirring new drama, keep your message short and neutral. You might say,

"Hey everyone, I'm taking a break from this chat for my own peace. Nothing personal."

That's enough. You don't owe a speech. If someone tries to guilt-trip you, remember: the people who value you will respect your boundaries.

Sometimes the bravest thing you can do is walk away quietly.

***

Rebuilding After a Rumor

Digital rumors spread like wildfire, and the aftermath can leave you feeling exposed or isolated. But even the biggest rumor loses power when you stop feeding it with attention.

One girl told me she went through this exact thing—a false story about her spread through group chats and stories. At first, she felt crushed, constantly checking who viewed her posts. Eventually, she deleted the apps for a few weeks. *"It felt like I was disappearing,"* she said, *"but really, I was just reclaiming my peace."*

When she returned, the drama had already burned out. The people who mattered listened to her side, and the ones who didn't had moved on. She slowly rebuilt her confidence, piece by piece.

Stepping back doesn't erase what happened, but it gives you room to remember who you are outside the noise.

***

Practical Wisdom for Next Time

Digital spaces can make communication tricky. Without tone or expression, messages can sound colder than intended. Jokes can look cruel in screenshots. And sometimes people act tougher behind screens than they ever would in person.

Before posting or replying, try this: imagine the person's face right in front of you. Would you still say it the same way?

If the answer's no, it's worth rephrasing—or not sending at all.

And when you see someone else being targeted, you can quietly show support. Send a kind DM to them about their latest post. Let them know they're not alone. Being the person who brings calm into chaos is its own kind of strength.

***

A Quiet Reminder

You are not the rumor. You are not the thread. You are not the screenshot.

You are a real, whole person who deserves kindness—even from yourself.

Digital drama will always come and go, but your peace, your integrity, and your voice are things no one can screenshot away.

So the next time you feel pulled into the storm, pause. Breathe. Step back. And remember: silence, self-respect, and time are often the most powerful comebacks there are.

***

SAYING "NO" WITHOUT THE GUILT TRIP

Saying no sounds simple, but it can feel like one of the hardest words in the world to say—especially to people you care about. You want to do the right thing, but the moment a friend says, *"Come on, it's no big deal,"* your stomach twists. You start wondering: Will they think I'm boring? Am I letting them down? Will I get left out next time?

It's completely normal to feel torn. The desire to belong is powerful—it's wired into all of us. But sometimes the need to fit in bumps up against your values, and that's when the real challenge begins.

Why "No" Feels So Risky

When you say no, you're not just turning down an activity—you're risking connection. At least, that's how it feels in the moment. Whether it's skipping class, joining gossip, or going to a party you're unsure about, saying no can feel like standing on a cliff between who you are and who others want you to be.

But here's the truth: protecting your peace will always be worth more than temporary approval.

The first few times you say no, it might feel awkward or scary. Your voice might shake. You might overthink your words. But every time you choose your values over pressure, you grow stronger inside. Boundaries aren't about pushing people away—they're about teaching others how to treat you.

You deserve friends who respect your "no" instead of punishing you for having one.

***

Simple Ways to Say No

Having a few go-to phrases ready makes it easier when your brain freezes under pressure. You could say something like,

"I care about you, but I'm not comfortable with that."

"Thanks for inviting me, but I'll pass this time."

"That's not really my thing, but I hope it's fun."

These sentences are short, kind, and firm. They don't attack anyone—they express your choice clearly. You're giving respect while expecting it back.

If someone keeps pushing, it's okay to repeat yourself calmly or change the subject. You don't owe a long explanation. A simple *"I'd rather not"* or *"Let's talk about something else"* is enough.

Good friends might tease a little or ask questions at first, but real ones will accept your boundaries. If they can't—if they pout, pressure, or guilt-trip you—it says more about the friendship than about your choice.

***

Assertive, Not Aggressive

There's a big difference between being assertive and being aggressive. Assertiveness is confidence with kindness—it protects both you and the friendship. Aggression usually stems from fear or anger and pushes people away.

> **Here's the difference:**
> If someone asks you to skip class, **assertiveness might sound like,**
> *"I'd rather not—I need to get my work done."*
> **Aggressive would sound like,**
> *"Why do you always want to break the rules? This is so stupid."*

The first answer is clear and calm; the second is defensive and judgmental. Assertiveness keeps the door open to mutual respect.

When you speak your truth with steadiness instead of shame, people notice. They may not say it out loud, but many quietly admire someone who can stand their ground with grace.

***

When Guilt Sneaks In

Even after you've said no, guilt might come knocking. You'll replay the conversation, wondering if you hurt their feelings or overreacted. That's normal—it's the people-pleaser part of your brain trying to protect you from rejection.

But guilt often shows up not because you did something wrong, but because you did something different. You broke an old pattern—choosing yourself first—and your mind is still catching up to the new normal.

When that guilt hits, pause and ask yourself:

Was I honest?

Was I respectful?

Did I stay true to what matters to me?

If the answer is yes, take a deep breath. You didn't fail—you succeeded. You practiced courage.

Sometimes, after the initial discomfort, relief follows. Freedom. Pride. A quiet voice whispering, I did it—I chose me.

You can even celebrate that small victory. Watch your favorite show, take a walk, write it down, or treat yourself to something tiny but meaningful. You deserve to feel good about standing your ground.

***

WHAT BOUNDARIES REALLY ARE

A lot of people think boundaries mean building walls, but they're actually the opposite. A boundary is a door—you choose when it's open and when it's closed.

You can let people in when it feels right and step back when you need space. It's not about control; it's about choice.

Friends who care about you might not love every boundary at first, but they'll respect them because they respect you. Suppose someone reacts with anger, manipulation, or guilt. In that case, that reaction is revealing—they're showing you how much they value control over connection.

Remember: it's okay to outgrow relationships that can't honor your boundaries.

> **Practicing Real-Life Scenarios**
> Picture this: your friends invite you to a party where you know there'll be drinking. You feel uneasy. Your instinct says no—but your heart worries they'll think you're lame.
> You can try something like,
> *"I'm gonna skip this one, but I hope you have fun. Let's hang out another time."*
> Or maybe someone starts gossiping about another friend and tries to pull you in. You could say,
> *"I don't feel right talking about them when they're not here."*

It might feel awkward at first, but awkward doesn't mean wrong. It just means you're stepping into integrity—and that's the kind of strength that lasts.

Every "no" that honors your values builds a kind of quiet confidence that doesn't need applause.

Journaling Moment

Think about a time you said no—even if it came out shaky or late. What did that moment reveal about what's important to you?

Write about how it felt before, during, and after. What changed in you once you stood by your decision? Did you feel freer, prouder, calmer? Did you notice who respected your choice—and who didn't?

Then ask yourself: What does saying no allow me to say yes to instead?

It could be peace of mind. Perhaps it's self-respect. It may be time for things that truly fill you up.

Every boundary honored is a message to yourself: *I matter, too.*

***

A Closing Reminder

Saying no doesn't make you cold, rude, or selfish. It makes it clear.

It means you know what you value and you're brave enough to protect it. And while not everyone will understand that right away, the right people—the ones who genuinely care—will.

They'll respect you for it. Some might even wish they had your courage.

Learning to say no is one of the quietest but strongest ways to build self-respect. Over time, it transforms your relationships from people-pleasing to real connection—where honesty, not fear, holds the friendship together.

And when you say yes, it'll finally mean something, because it'll come from choice, not pressure.

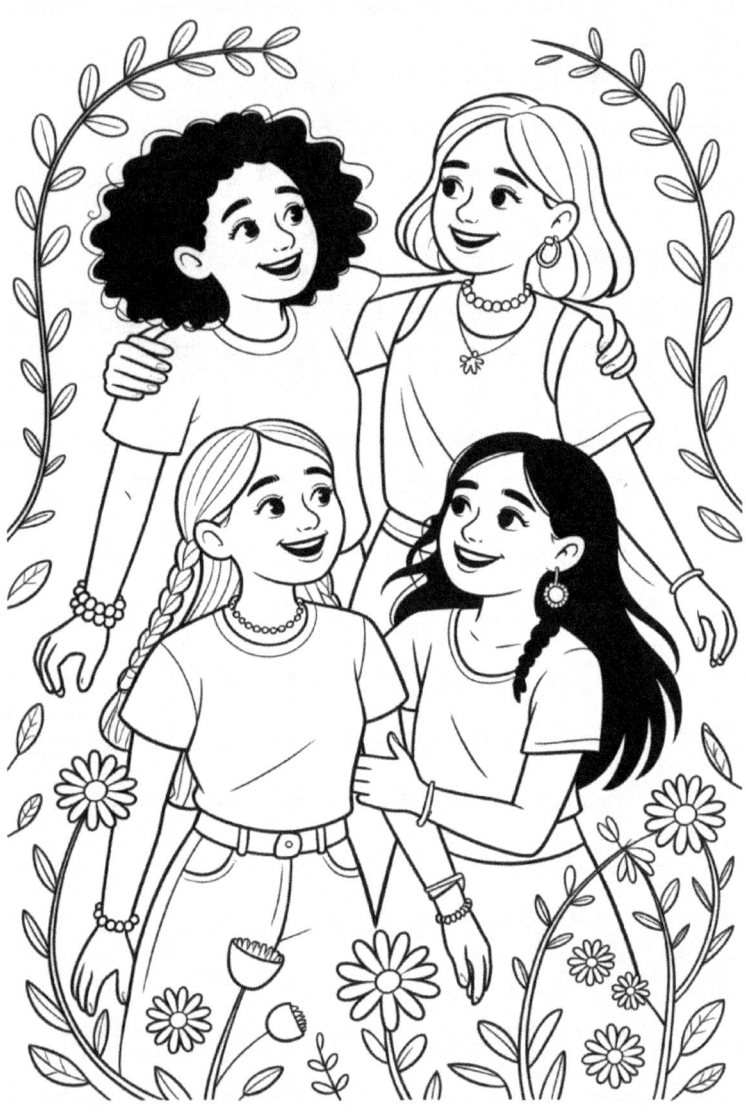

Chapter 3

Social Media Survival

Curating a Feed That Feeds You

It's a scenario many of us can relate to: you wake up, grab your phone, and are immediately bombarded with a stream of seemingly perfect moments. A friend is on a sunrise run, another's hair looks like it's straight out of a commercial, and a classmate is sharing photos from a concert you didn't even know was happening. It's a constant reel of everyone else seemingly living their best life, while you're still untangling yesterday's homework and bedhead.

But here's the secret: what you're seeing isn't real life—it's a highlight reel. Understanding this can be a powerful tool in your social media survival kit, relieving you from the pressure of unrealistic comparisons.

Social media platforms are built for showing the best parts—the smiles, the wins, the celebrations—not the mess behind them. You rarely see the meltdowns, the bad lighting, or the moments that didn't cut. It's like watching a movie trailer that skips all the boring, complicated, human parts of the story.

And yet, when you're scrolling half-awake in your room, it's easy to forget that. Your brain, wired to compare, starts whispering, *Why can't my life look like that? Why can't I look like that?*

Even when you know those images are filtered and edited, it can still sting. That's because comparison isn't just about logic—it's emotional.

WHEN COMPARISON STARTS QUIETLY

You might not even notice it at first. It begins with small thoughts: *I wish my skin looked that clear. Her room's so aesthetic. She always seems so confident.* Before long, the quiet envy turns into a heavier feeling—like your everyday life isn't enough.

This isn't about jealousy; it's about how your brain reacts to repetition. Seeing hundreds of "perfect" images every day trains your mind to expect that perfection from yourself. Over time, it can chip away at how you see your body, your achievements, even your worth.

Psychologists call it social comparison, and studies show it can raise anxiety and lower self-esteem—especially for teen girls. The constant feed of flawless photos and curated smiles makes it harder to remember that everyone's highlight reel leaves out their real life.

Even the people who look effortlessly confident online have their bad days—they don't post them. That candid TikTok dance? It probably took twenty tries. That "chill beach day" photo? Maybe it happened right after an argument.

One girl shared that her "best birthday ever" picture—complete with balloons, cake, and a perfect smile—was taken minutes before she cried in the bathroom because she felt left out of her own party.

***

The Hidden Truth Behind the Feed

The truth is, every post has a story you don't see. The smiling beach photo might have been snapped after hours of frustration about what to wear. The flawless selfie could be hiding twenty retakes and a heavy filter. The influencer who "woke up like this" might have spent half an hour fixing their hair and lighting.

You're not broken for forgetting that sometimes. The internet was designed to make perfection look effortless—and effort invisible.

Recognizing this can empower you to take control of your social media experience. Next time you find yourself comparing, pause and ask yourself: What might be happening outside the frame? Maybe that friend is posting more because they're lonely. Perhaps the person who seems fearless is struggling with something they haven't shared. Remembering that every photo is just one second of someone's life helps loosen the grip of comparisons.

You can even write it down. Pick a post that made you feel "less than," and jot down what could be unseen—the emotions, the retakes, the reality behind the picture. Imagining the whole scene helps you remember that no one's life is perfectly polished.

***

Refocusing on What's Real

When comparison starts to steal your joy, gently bring your focus back to your own world—the one that's actually happening around you. This practice can help you feel more grounded and present in your own life. Try this: at the start or end of your day, list three small things you genuinely appreciate. They don't have to be huge. Maybe it's a snack that hit the spot, a text that made you laugh, or that moment when the sky looked beautiful for no reason.

It's a slight shift, but it's powerful. Gratitude pulls your attention out of the illusion and back into your reality—the place where real connection, not performance, lives.

Your life might not look like someone else's feed, but it's full of tiny, beautiful things you can actually touch and feel.

Curating a Feed That Feeds You

Your feed should be like a playlist for your mental health—curated with intention. You get to choose what voices fill your screen and how they make you feel.

Follow creators who remind you that life is messy, that growth takes time, and that it's okay to be human. There are people out there who post about failure, anxiety, breakouts, and bad days—and somehow, their honesty feels like a deep breath.

Unfollow or mute accounts that drain your energy. If scrolling someone's page leaves you tense, comparing, or sad, it's okay to take a break. Protecting your mental space is more important than keeping up appearances.

One student told me she started unfollowing influencers who made her feel "not enough" and replaced them with artists, activists, and creators who shared behind-the-scenes reality. *"It felt weird at first,"* she said, *"like I was leaving the cool crowd. But then I started liking my own life again."*

***

POSTING WITH PURPOSE

You can also be part of changing the culture. Try posting one real moment—not a highlight, not an edited masterpiece, just something true: your messy desk, your goofy grin, your unfiltered morning.

The first time might feel vulnerable. But the response might surprise you—people often crave authenticity more than perfection. Your honesty permits them to be honest, too.

The more you share what's real, the more space you create for others to breathe.

Behind-the-Scenes Reality Check

Here's a simple exercise you can try tonight: pick a photo on your feed or camera roll that looks 'perfect.' Then, in a notebook or notes app, write what happened just before and after that shot.

This exercise can help you see the reality behind the 'perfect' posts and foster a healthier relationship with your social media feed. Were you nervous? Rushed? Excited? Tired? Did you take twenty versions before posting one? Did anything go wrong?

Naming what was happening behind the photo helps you remember that even your own posts have layers others don't see. You're not the only one with a "real life" behind the filter.

As you scroll, pay attention to how your body feels. Does this post make you smile, laugh, or feel inspired? Keep it. Does it tighten your chest or spark self-doubt? Mute it, unfollow it, or take a break from it.

You are allowed to protect your peace—even from pixels.

***

The Power of Intentional Scrolling

Every swipe, like, and comment affects how you feel. Instead of letting the algorithm decide for you, make conscious choices.

Think of your feed like your mental diet. If all you consume are filtered lives, you'll start craving perfection that doesn't exist. But if you fill your feed with honesty, creativity, and kindness, you'll start feeling more grounded in your own story.

Used thoughtfully, social media can connect you to real people and ideas that truly feed your soul. You can find art that inspires you, creators who make you laugh, or communities that remind you you're not alone.

But it starts with intention—choosing what adds light and muting what dims it.

***

Reclaiming the Joy of Being Real

The next time you scroll and feel the sting of comparison, pause and remind yourself: *I'm looking at a highlight reel, not a whole movie.*

Perfection might get likes, but authenticity builds connection—and that's what truly lasts.

Your worth isn't measured in followers, filters, or hearts. It's measured in how fully you show up as yourself—in how you treat people, how you learn, how you keep going.

You don't need to match anyone's highlight reel. Your everyday, imperfect, beautiful life is already enough.

When you fill your feed with truth, gratitude, and laughter, you stop chasing someone else's story and start living your own. And that's the kind of content worth sharing.

VIBE-CHECKING YOUR FEED FOR TOXIC ENERGY

Every scroll shapes how you see yourself and the world. Some posts make you smile or spark an idea; others quietly drain you, leaving behind an uneasy feeling you can't name. It's easy to shrug it off as "just social media," but your feed has absolute power over your mood, your confidence, and even your sense of who you are.

Apparent negativity—mean comments, gossip, shaming memes—is easy to spot. The trickier kind hides behind glossy filters and "positive" captions. Maybe it's a friend's constant humble-bragging, an influencer's impossible morning routine, or a string of "perfect" updates that make your own life feel dull by comparison. These small jabs of envy or self-doubt pile up quietly until you notice your energy fading.

***

Listening to Your Body While You Scroll

Your body is usually the first to know when something online feels off. Notice how you react as you scroll: does your chest tighten, your shoulders hunch, or your mind start racing? Do you feel a flicker of jealousy, irritation, or that familiar "I'm not enough" feeling creeping in?

If certain posts always leave you tense or deflated, it's time for a vibe-check. Social platforms are designed to stir emotion—likes, streaks, notifications—all of it pulls at your need for validation. But you don't have to hand them your peace of mind.

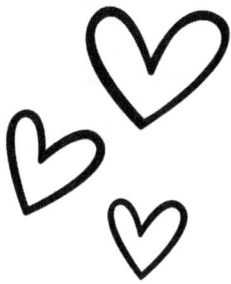

Try a quick self-check after a scroll session:

- Did this content lift my confidence or shrink it?

- Am I feeling inspired or drained?

- Did I smile, or did my mood drop a little?

- Do I actually want to connect with this person, or do I feel worse after seeing their life?

When the answer leans toward "tired" or "less than," that's a cue to protect your space.

***

Clearing the Hidden Clutter

Cleaning your feed is like cleaning your room—you often don't realize how much clutter is stressing you out until it's gone. If certain accounts regularly stir anxiety or comparison, give yourself permission to mute, unfollow, or restrict them. Your mental health matters more than digital politeness.

Worried it'll cause drama? Muting is a gentle middle ground. You'll stay connected, but their posts disappear from your feed. And if someone ever asks, it's completely fine to say, *"I'm taking a little step back from social media for my mental health."* Most people understand—some will even relate.

One reader told me she followed a fitness influencer for months before realizing she dreaded opening the app. *"Every post made me feel like I wasn't doing enough,"* she said. When she finally unfollowed those accounts and replaced them with body-positive creators who celebrated strength and self-acceptance, she said she could breathe again.

Your peace is worth a quiet unfollow.

From One-Time Clean to Digital Ritual

You've already cleared the clutter—now it's time to keep your space light. Think of this as a quick weekly or monthly "feed reset." It doesn't take long, but it can make a big difference.

Set aside ten quiet minutes, sit somewhere calm, and open your following list. Scroll slowly and ask yourself:

Does this bring me positivity, learning, laughter, relaxation, or real connection?

Do I feel lighter or heavier after seeing their posts?

If the answer leans toward 'heavier, 'feel the freedom in letting it go. No guilt. No explanations. Just the lightness of a digital burden lifted.

Then, refill your feed with energy that inspires you—an artist you admire, a friend who makes you laugh, or a page that reminds you to breathe. The goal isn't more followers; it's the joy of discovering better energy.

One girl shared how a simple "feed cleanse" changed her mood: *"I didn't realize how many posts were making me anxious until I deleted them. My screen time went down, my focus improved, and I started liking social media again."*

This is what a proper digital reset looks like—gentle, intentional, freeing.

You deserve to open your phone and see things that build you up, not wear you down. It's your digital space, and you have the power to curate it for your well-being.

***

Creating a "Happy Feed"

Once you've made feed resets a habit, fill that space with accounts that truly nourish you. Think of it as planting a new garden after pulling weeds.

Look for creators who show both their wins and their rough days—artists sharing behind-the-scenes sketches, students talking honestly about burnout, athletes posting about progress rather than perfection. Follow pages that connect you with hobbies you love or that remind you of your values: mental health, kindness, curiosity, creativity, faith—whatever centers you.

You can even make a private collection of "feel-good" posts to revisit when you need a lift. Save funny memes, encouraging quotes, or the posts that make you exhale and think, *Oh good, it's not just me.*

Over time, your feed can become a space that recharges you rather than drains you—a reflection of who you're becoming, not who you think you need to be.

***

A Gentle Four-Step Refresh

If you like having a small structure to follow, try this rhythm next time your feed feels heavy:

Find your calm spot. Sit somewhere quiet—maybe your bed, a park bench, or your favorite corner of the couch.

Scroll slowly and notice. As you review who you follow, listen to your gut more than your guilt.

Release what feels wrong. Unfollow, mute, or hide anything that spikes stress or dulls your joy.

Add what feels right. Refill your feed with people, ideas, and pages that make you feel creative, grounded, or genuinely connected.

It's not about perfection; it's about alignment.

***

Why It Matters

Every post you see leaves a small fingerprint on your thoughts. Over time, those impressions add up. A feed full of impossible beauty standards and fake positivity can make even confident people question themselves. But a feed full of authenticity and compassion reminds you that life doesn't have to be polished to be beautiful.

You deserve to open your phone and see things that build you up, not wear you down.

Social media doesn't have to be a constant competition. It can be a gallery of what inspires you—a place to celebrate your growth, not chase someone else's approval.

***

Your Feed, Your Energy

Imagine your feed as a mirror. What do you want it to reflect to you? Pressure, comparison, or peace?

When you choose accounts that reflect your values, your feed starts to feel like home again. You'll scroll and see reminders of kindness, humor, and creativity—the things that actually feed your spirit.

That's what curating your space is all about: empowering yourself to protect your energy so that your digital world supports your real one. And when your online life begins to echo your true self—messy, curious, alive—you'll notice the difference everywhere else too. Your confidence grows quieter and steadier. Your comparisons fade. Your joy expands, inspiring a brighter offline world. You don't have to delete social media to find peace. You have to decide what deserves space on your screen—and in your mind.

***

A Closing Reflection

Take one last look at your feed today. See it not as something happening to you, but something you have power over.

This isn't about pretending everything's perfect; it's about creating an environment that protects your light and reflects who you're becoming.

You deserve a feed that feels like breathing room—a digital reflection of your worth, your curiosity, and your peace.

Because when your online world feels right, your offline world starts to glow a little brighter too.

***

CYBERBULLYING SOS — WHAT TO DO WHEN THE HATE IS ONLINE

Cyberbullying isn't just "someone being mean." It's a repeated, targeted attack through your phone or computer meant to make you feel small, scared, or ashamed. It can show up in dozens of ways — nasty direct messages, cruel comments, being excluded from group chats, or seeing your name turned into a meme. Sometimes it's obvious, like insults filling your DMs. Other times, it's sneaky: inside jokes that cut deep, private photos shared without permission, or silence from people who used to be your friends.

Even one hateful message can stick with you. When it happens over and over, it can start to feel like there's no safe place to escape.

***

First Things First: You Don't Have to Face It Alone

If you're being targeted online, please know this: you're not overreacting, and you don't have to "just ignore it." You deserve safety — even on a screen. You are not alone in this struggle.

The most important thing is to protect yourself before trying to fix anything.

Start by **not responding** to the person or group attacking you. That can be incredibly hard, especially when you want to defend yourself or clap back. But most bullies crave a reaction — that's what keeps them going. Choosing silence is not weakness; it's a strategy.

Next, **block or mute** the person immediately. Don't wait to see if they'll stop. On most platforms, blocking prevents them from messaging or tagging you again. If the bullying happens in a group chat, mute or leave it altogether.

Every tap that reclaims your peace is an act of strength.

***

Save the Evidence — Even When It Hurts to Look

When something cruel happens online, your first instinct might be to delete it — you want it gone. But saving evidence can protect you later.

Take **screenshots** of every mean comment, DM, meme, or post. Make sure the username, date, and time are visible. You can store them in a hidden folder or email them to yourself. That way, if things continue or escalate, you have proof.

Think of it as collecting facts, not feelings. You're not keeping the hate; you're keeping the truth.

***

Reach Out for Backup

Bullying feeds on silence. The moment you tell someone, the situation starts to lose power.

Find one trusted person — a parent, counselor, teacher, coach, or even a friend's older sibling — and let them know what's happening. You don't have to have all the words figured out. You could start with something as simple as, *"I'm getting mean messages online and I need help."*

You don't need to share every screenshot right away. Just open the door.

Adults and school staff can help you decide what to do next — whether that's reporting the behavior to the platform, contacting a teacher, or involving law enforcement if it crosses into threats or harassment.

Remember: asking for help isn't tattling or weak. It's taking control.

***

Use the Tools at Your Fingertips

Every social platform has tools to help you protect yourself. You have to know where to find them.

On **Instagram**, tap the three dots next to a post or a DM, then select *"Report"* or *"Block."* You can also filter who can comment or message you under *Settings → Privacy.*

On **TikTok**, long-press a comment to report or delete it and block the user.

On **Snapchat**, press and hold on the username, then choose *"Report"* or *"Block."* You can also turn off who's allowed to send you Snaps or view your stories.

Each app lets you take back some control. After reporting, most platforms send a confirmation email or message—keep that too as part of your record.

If you're unsure how to navigate any of this, ask a trusted adult to sit beside you while you do it. Sometimes just having someone nearby helps you breathe easier.

***

Real Story: How One Girl Took Her Power Back

One teen told me that after switching schools, she began getting anonymous DMs almost every night. At first, she ignored them, hoping they'd stop. Instead, they got worse — messages about her clothes, her voice, even her family.

Finally, she told her aunt. Together, they took screenshots, saved every message, and brought them to the school counselor. Her aunt also helped her adjust her privacy settings and block fake accounts.

Then she made a private group chat with a few friends who'd always had her back. They checked in daily — not about the bullies, but about ordinary life, jokes, schoolwork, plans for the weekend. *"It reminded me,"* she said, *"that not everyone online is cruel. My real friends still saw me."*

That small circle became her safe zone — a digital home base filled with kindness instead of chaos.

***

If You See Someone Being Targeted

Even if you're not the one being bullied, what you do matters more than you might realize. Online cruelty spreads quickly, but so does kindness — it just needs someone brave enough to start it.

> **If you see cyberbullying happen:**
> Don't engage with the hate. Don't like, share, or comment on cruel posts, even to say "stop." Every click gives the content more attention.
> Instead, quietly message the person being targeted. It can be as simple as, *"I saw what's happening. I'm here if you need someone."*
> Use the app's tools to report the post or account.
> If what you're seeing includes threats, personal info leaks, or stalking, tell an adult right away — even if it's not directed at you.

Standing by your values might cost you "clout," but it strengthens something far more important — your integrity.

The Power of an Ally

Sometimes, being the one person who doesn't join in can change everything. One quiet message can feel like a lifeline to someone drowning in cruelty.

If you're unsure what to say, try:

"I know that post isn't fair to you."

"You don't deserve that."

"I reported it. You're not alone."

Even if they never reply, your kindness lands. It reminds them that not everyone has turned away.

You don't have to fight the bully to make an impact; sometimes the bravest act is choosing not to add to the noise.

***

Rebuilding After Online Hate

When the messages finally stop, you might expect relief—but the emotions often linger. Hurtful words have a way of echoing in your head long after they disappear from your screen.

It helps to take a break from your phone entirely for a few days. Spend time offline doing things that bring you back to yourself — walking, journaling, baking, drawing, praying, listening to music that steadies you.

You might even make a "kindness folder" on your phone — screenshots of encouraging messages, funny memes, compliments, or quotes that lift you. When the world feels cruel, open it. Remind yourself that goodness still exists — and that you're part of it.

Suppose the pain feels too heavy or the harassment has shaken your confidence deeply. In that case, it's okay to ask for professional support. Talking to a counselor or therapist doesn't mean you're broken; it means you're healing intentionally.

A Final Word About Worth

Cyberbullying can make you question who you are. But no amount of online hate can erase your worth or your voice.

Every time you block, report, save proof, or reach out for help, you're choosing courage. Every time you refuse to mirror cruelty, you're choosing strength.

The internet can be loud and cruel, but it can also be kind — and you have power in shaping which version you participate in.

You don't have to fight every battle, and you don't have to handle the pain alone. Protect your peace. Lean on your people. And remember: the screen may feel endless, but it's not the whole world.

Beyond it, there's still sunlight, laughter, music, and genuine connection waiting for you. That's the world that deserves your energy.

***

UNPLUG, UNFOLLOW, UNWIND — CREATING A HEALTHIER DIGITAL ROUTINE

You don't have to be glued to your phone to belong.

You don't have to check every notification or story to matter.

Taking time away from your screen isn't weird—it's healthy. In fact, it might be one of the kindest things you can do for yourself. That constant ping, the endless scroll, the tiny urge to "just check one more thing"—it all adds up. It fills your head with noise and steals quiet moments that could've been laughter, stillness, or creativity.

Skipping a post or staying offline for a few hours won't make you invisible. It might actually help you feel *seen* again—by yourself.

***

What Unplugging Really Means

A lot of phone anxiety comes from the pressure always to be reachable, to stay "in the loop." We tell ourselves that if we step away, we'll miss something important. But here's the twist: unplugging doesn't disconnect you—it reconnects you.

When you step back from your screen, life comes into focus again. You notice the warmth of sunlight through your window, the sound of your dog breathing beside you, the way your favorite song sounds when you're not distracted by another tab or text. You catch up with a friend face-to-face and realize that real laughter doesn't need likes or filters to count.

What you're really gaining isn't distance from the world—it's closeness to the parts that matter most.

***

Setting Boundaries With Your Phone

Think of technology boundaries the same way you'd think of healthy boundaries with people. It's not about cutting anyone off—it's about deciding what's suitable for your peace of mind.

Start small.

Your phone already has built-in tools to help. Try setting daily time limits for apps that eat up your hours—Instagram, TikTok, or YouTube. When the reminder pops up, pause for just five seconds and ask: *Is scrolling what I really want right now? Or am I just filling space?*

Make phone-free zones part of your day.

Put your phone away after 9 p.m. and give your brain time to unwind before bed. Keep it off your nightstand so your first moments in the morning belong to you, not your feed. Please leave it in your bag during lunch or dinner so you can taste your food and really talk.

Even one tiny change—like not checking notifications before school—can shift the tone of your entire day.

***

Replacing the Scroll With Real Joy

If being offline feels strange at first, that's normal. You're breaking a habit ingrained in your routine. But the beautiful part is: you get to replace it with something better.

Grab a sketchbook and doodle without worrying if it's "good." Journal about your day, your mood, or your dreams—no one else has to read it. Put on a playlist that matches your energy and sing out loud while you get ready.

Or try what one reader called her "main character moments." She'd pick something creative to do offline—baking, learning a TikTok dance without posting it, or writing a story just for fun. It reminded her that her life didn't need an audience to matter.

Every time you do something offline that fills you up, you remind yourself that your life is *yours*—not a performance.

What You Notice When You Step Away

After you take a break, even a short one, notice how you feel. Sometimes the change is subtle—maybe you fall asleep faster or feel less anxious at bedtime. Other times it's more obvious: you might laugh louder, focus better, or realize how much time opens up when your hand isn't glued to your phone.

One girl told me that after putting her phone away for just an afternoon, she ended up painting for the first time in years. Another said she felt "like a person again" after spending a weekend camping without Wi-Fi.

These breaks don't mean you're anti-social; they tell you you're finally letting your own thoughts breathe.

***

A Simple Challenge: 24 Hours Offline

If you're up for it, try a 24-hour social media break—one full day.

Put your phone somewhere safe—like a drawer, a backpack, wherever—and go about your life. The first few hours might feel strange, even itchy, like you're missing a limb. But after a while, something shifts. You might notice you're calmer. Time stretches. Your brain feels clearer.

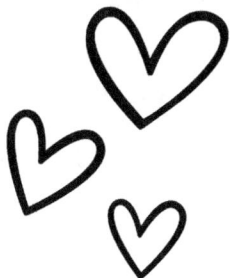

Then, write about it.

Ask yourself:

- What did I actually miss?

- What did I notice, or what did I do instead?

- Did my mood change?

You might be surprised by how much lighter you feel when your mind isn't buzzing with other people's lives.

If 24 hours feels too long, start smaller. One hour a day. Then two. Build up slowly.

***

Making It Fun — Not a Punishment

You can even make unplugging a game. Invite a friend to join you. Have a "digital detox" movie night where everyone drops their phones in a basket. Or turn it into a mini challenge: who can last the longest without checking notifications? The winner gets bragging rights—or maybe just the satisfaction of remembering what freedom feels like.

Celebrate your wins, no matter how small. You could have finished a book. Maybe you went outside just because. Perhaps you cooked dinner with your family or laughed until your stomach hurt.

Those moments might not get likes, but they fill you up in ways a screen never could.

Listening to Your Emotions — Not the Apps

Part of building a healthier digital routine is tuning back in to what *you* feel, rather than what your phone tells you to feel. Apps are designed to pull you in with endless new content. But your emotions are clues—pay attention to them.

If you start scrolling and feel anxious, bored, or numb, pause.

Ask yourself: *What am I really looking for right now?*

Sometimes it's a distraction. Sometimes it's comfort. Sometimes it's a connection. But those needs can often be met better offline—with a walk, a nap, a call to a real friend, or just a quiet moment alone.

You have every right to protect your mental space from the pull of algorithms.

***

Sharing the Break

Once you've felt the calm of being offline, please share it. Tell a friend how freeing it was to not worry about likes or comments for a while. Please encourage them to try a mini digital detox of their own. You might inspire someone who didn't realize how much social media was weighing them down.

Try this together: spend one afternoon without phones: no scrolling, no filming, no updates. Just hang out. Cook, walk, paint, or talk. You'll discover that honest conversations are easier when nobody's half-listening through a screen.

Offline time can actually deepen friendships because you're fully present. It's not about escaping the internet—it's about coming home to yourself.

***

Making Balance Your Goal

A healthier digital life isn't about strict rules or guilt. It's about balance—the kind that makes your phone a tool, not a trap.

You're allowed to set limits, to step back, to log off when you need peace. The world won't forget you. Your friends will still be there. What changes is that *you* return calmer, stronger, and more centered.

Technology should work for you, not the other way around.

***

A Closing Reflection

When you close your apps for a little while, what you open instead is space—space for laughter, creativity, and genuine connection. You get to decide when and how you engage, rather than letting your phone determine for you.

You're not missing out when you unplug. You're tuning in—to your mind, your body, your values, and your real life.

Each break, no matter how short, is a reminder: you are more than your notifications. You are allowed to rest, to breathe, to live outside the feed.

Because when you come back online, you'll bring more of your true self with you—and that's the version the world most needs to see.

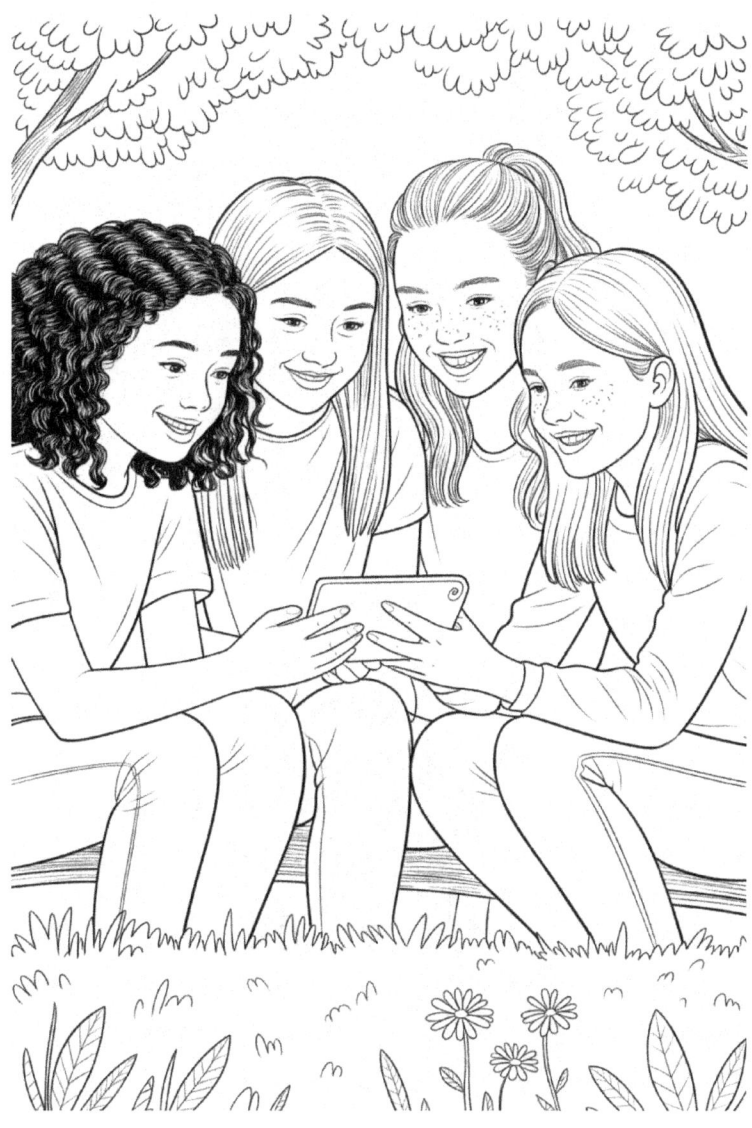

***

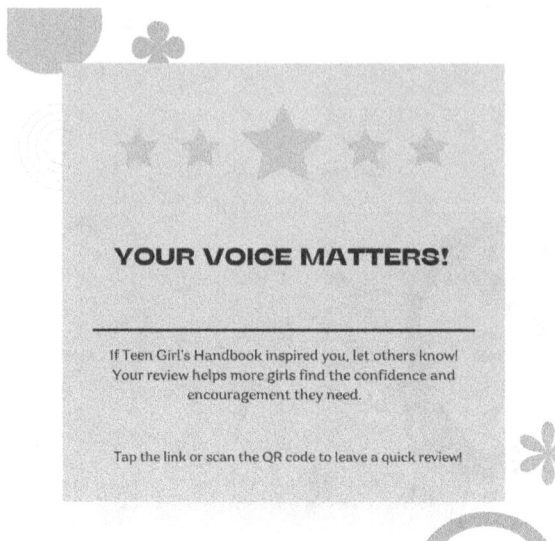

YOUR VOICE MATTERS!

If Teen Girl's Handbook inspired you, let others know!
Your review helps more girls find the confidence and
encouragement they need.

Tap the link or scan the QR code to leave a quick review!

Scan the QR code to leave your review.

***

Chapter 4

Stress Less

Real Tools for Academic Pressure and Overwhelm

P icture this: you're sitting at your desk, staring at a blank Google Doc that feels like it's mocking you. The cursor blinks. You tell yourself you'll check one more text or watch one quick video before you start. Ten minutes pass. Then twenty. Suddenly, the night feels shorter, the work feels heavier, and that familiar pit forms in your stomach.

That's procrastination.

Remember, almost everyone does it—especially students who *care* about doing things well. It's not laziness or lack of discipline. More often, it's fear. Fear of not doing it perfectly. Fear of failing. Fear of starting something big and not knowing how it will go.

Procrastination is your brain's way of coping with fear. It seeks quick relief through distractions like scrolling through memes, taking extended snack breaks, or watching videos. Remember, you're not broken; you're just trying to escape the pressure that fear brings.

***

PROCRASTINATION PANIC: WHY IT HAPPENS

Procrastination often hides behind perfectionism. That little voice says, *"If I can't do this perfectly, why even start?"* or *"What if I mess up and everyone realizes I'm not as smart as they think?"*

So instead of starting, you freeze. You think, *"I'll do it later when I feel ready."* But "later" rarely comes with more motivation—just more guilt. And guilt makes the mountain look even taller.

Many teen girls fall into this exact pattern because they care deeply about grades, expectations, and not letting anyone down. Research shows that teens are more likely to procrastinate when a task feels too big, too vague, or too closely tied to their self-worth. It's like your brain decides: *If success equals being good enough, failure must mean I'm not.* So, to avoid that pain, you delay starting at all.

Here's a positive perspective: procrastination isn't a permanent habit. It's a signal from your brain, saying, *"I feel overwhelmed and need a smaller first step."* It's an opportunity to break tasks into manageable chunks and take the first step towards progress.

***

Shrinking the Mountain

When something feels impossible, shrink it until it no longer does.

Try the **five-minute rule**. Tell yourself, "I'll just do this for five minutes." That's it. Set a timer, open the assignment, and start—even if you only outline the first sentence or skim a few notes. Starting is the most challenging part because it breaks the mental wall between *thinking about doing something* and *actually doing it.*

Most of the time, once you begin, you'll find the momentum to keep going. But even if you stop at five minutes, you've already shifted from stuck to started—and that matters.

***

Breaking Tasks Into Tiny Wins

Big goals feel less scary when you turn them into small, doable actions. Instead of writing "Finish history paper" on your to-do list (which sounds like a nightmare), break it down into manageable steps:

- Choose a topic

- Write a one-sentence thesis

- Find one reliable source

- Draft one paragraph

- Revisit the next day to edit

Each small checkmark is a mini confidence boost. It's proof you're moving forward. Small steps also quiet the perfectionist voice because they don't feel high-stakes—they feel manageable.

One student told me she renamed her to-do list "Tiny Victories" to make it feel less intimidating. The change worked—every time she crossed off a micro-task, she felt a rush of progress instead of dread.

***

Finding Focus That Feels Good

If distractions keep winning, try switching up your space or using tools that make focus easier:

Change your environment. Move to a quiet corner of the library, a cozy café, or even the floor by your window. Sometimes a new spot resets your brain.

Play background music. Lo-fi, instrumental, or movie soundtracks can block noise without distracting you with lyrics.

Try the Pomodoro method. Work for 25 minutes, take a 5-minute break, repeat 4 times, then take a more extended break. It turns studying into a rhythm instead of a marathon.

Find a "body double." Work side-by-side with a friend—either in person or on a quiet video call. You don't have to talk; just knowing someone else is working helps keep you accountable.

Think of focus as something you can *design,* not just something you can force.

Interactive Exercise — The Break-It-Down Worksheet

- Grab a piece of paper, your Notes app, or your planner. Write your most significant current assignment at the top—maybe that essay, science project, or book report you've been avoiding.

- Now, list every single step you can think of to complete it:

- **brainstorm → outline → gather sources → draft → revise → proofread → format.**

- Assign one or two of those micro-tasks to each day this week. Each time you finish one, cross it off and celebrate. Those small completions add up faster than you think.

Handling the Crash Without Shame

Everyone slips. You might lose a day (or a few) to procrastination and panic. The worst thing you can do is pile guilt on top of stress.

Your inner critic might start shouting: *"You're so lazy!" "You'll never catch up!"*

But that voice isn't telling the truth—it's telling the story of someone scared.

Try answering back gently, the way you'd comfort a friend:

"It's okay. Everyone struggles with this sometimes."

"I can start again. I don't have to be perfect—just present."

Remember, self-compassion resets your brain faster than self-blame ever will.

When you catch yourself spiraling, pause for a reset ritual:

Stretch your body

Take a slow breath by a window

Drink water

Then, open your planner and choose *one small thing* to do next

You don't have to do it all tonight. You have to do one thing.

***

Learning From the Pause

Procrastination can actually teach you something—about what overwhelms you, what you avoid, and where your fear hides.

Ask yourself:

What exactly am I avoiding? The task—or how it makes me feel?

Am I trying to protect myself from failure or embarrassment?

What would happen if I let go of "perfect" and aimed for "done"?

Reflecting turns avoidance into awareness. And awareness gives you control.

Journaling Prompt

- *When I procrastinate, what does my inner critic say?*

- *How could I answer back with kindness, logic, or humor?*

Write both voices in your journal—the critic and the calm friend who replies. Notice what changes when you speak to yourself with compassion instead of judgment.

Even if you only write a few sentences, it helps you recognize that inner conversation for what it is—a dialogue you get to rewrite.

***

Redefining Success

Fast doesn't equal successful. Perfect doesn't equal proud.

Progress is what matters—steady, real, human progress. Every time you take a small step forward, even after getting stuck, you're proving to yourself that effort counts more than fear.

One girl told me she used to cry over every paper she turned in late. Then she started using a mantra: *"Done is better than perfect."* She said it out loud every time she submitted something that wasn't flawless—and her grades didn't fall. But her stress did.

You don't have to hustle to exhaustion to prove your worth.

You're already enough, even when you work slowly, even when you start late, even when you're learning as you go.

***

A Closing Thought

Procrastination doesn't mean you're bad at managing time—it means you're human. It means you care. It means your brain sometimes needs gentleness before it can move.

Each small choice to begin, each moment you show up even halfway, chips away at that heavy feeling of stuckness.

You don't have to conquer the whole mountain tonight.

Just take one brave step.

That's how every climb begins.

***

TEST ANXIETY TOOLKIT — CALM-DOWN RITUALS THAT ACTUALLY WORK

First, take a breath.

You're not broken because you get nervous before a test.

Test anxiety doesn't mean you're unprepared or inadequate at school. It's just your brain's way of saying, *"This matters to me."* When something feels important, your body reacts as if it's in danger—even if it's just a math quiz or essay prompt.

For some, anxiety shows up physically: a churning stomach, clammy hands, shaky legs, a racing heart, or a lump in the throat that makes it hard to swallow. For others, it's mental: your thoughts go blank, your pulse pounds in your ears, or your mind spirals into worst-case scenarios. You might even feel like crying, though you're not sure why.

These reactions are *normal*. They are signs that your nervous system is trying to protect you. Instead of fighting them, learn to listen. When you treat anxiety as information instead of a failure, it loses some of its power.

***

Quick Calm Rituals for Before or During a Test

If you've got only a few minutes to spare, try one of these grounding techniques. They don't require apps, special spaces, or complicated steps—just you, your breath, and a bit of focus.

1. The 4–7–8 Breath

Inhale through your nose for four seconds. Hold for seven. Exhale slowly through your mouth for eight. Repeat three times.

It may sound simple, but this slows your pulse, clears the mental fog, and signals your body that you're safe.

2. Visualization

Close your eyes for a moment and picture yourself walking into the test, calm and steady. Imagine flipping through the pages, remembering what you studied, writing confidently, and finishing with relief. Visualization tricks your brain into believing that calm is possible—because it is.

3. Music Reset

Before studying or walking into school, listen to a short playlist that sets your tone. Some teens find peace in quiet lo-fi or piano tracks; others focus better with upbeat songs that energize them. Choose what steadies you—not what distracts you.

***

Taming the Mind Spiral

Anxiety feeds off "what ifs."

What if I blank? What if I fail? What if everyone else finishes before me?

You can stop that spiral by grounding your thoughts in logic and self-kindness.

Grab a piece of paper or the notes app on your phone and write out three questions:

What's the absolute worst that could happen?

What's most likely to happen?

If it doesn't go well, what will I do next?

When you answer honestly, you usually see the pattern—your fears exaggerate the outcome, but the reality is manageable. You won't "ruin your life" if one test goes wrong. You'll recover, learn, and move on.

Then, replace the anxious narrative with affirmations that remind your brain what's true:

"A test is a snapshot, not my whole story."

"One grade doesn't decide my future."

"I know more than I think I do."

It might feel awkward at first, but repetition works. Over time, your brain learns that calm is possible—even in high-stress moments.

***

BUILDING A SCHOOL–LIFE BALANCE THAT FEELS RIGHT FOR YOU

Trying to do everything—ace every test, join every club, keep every plan—is a straight path to burnout. You might not even notice it happening at first. It starts as pride in being busy, or that rush you get from checking things off your list. But soon, your schedule starts running you instead of the other way around.

Take a step back and look at the big picture.

Grab a notebook and write down all your commitments: classes, sports, clubs, part-time jobs, hobbies, volunteer work, and social plans. Then, sort them into three columns:

> **Must-dos:** things that are nonnegotiable—like certain classes or responsibilities.
> **Want-to-dos:** things that bring you joy, meaning, or peace.
> **Energy vampires:** tasks, groups, or people that drain your energy or fill you with dread.

When you see everything laid out, it becomes easier to spot what's taking too much of you and what's actually giving something back. Balance doesn't come from doing everything—it comes from choosing what deserves your energy.

This exercise isn't selfish—it's honest. A club you loved last year might feel like a chore now. You might have joined a team because your friends did, but now you dread practice. Or maybe Sunday dinner with family is secretly the highlight of your week, even if it means missing something else.

Labeling your energy vampires doesn't mean cutting them out completely; it just helps you see where your time and energy might be leaking away.

***

Letting "Good Enough" Be Enough

Perfection sounds noble, but it's exhausting.

Not every project or quiz needs to be flawless. Sometimes a B-minus means you got a whole night's sleep, spent an hour laughing with friends, or finally took a deep breath. That's not failure—that's balance.

Learning to accept "good enough" is a quiet kind of strength. It's knowing when to give 100% and when to protect your energy for things that fill you up.

One student told me, *"The day I stopped aiming for perfect, I actually started enjoying school again."* She discovered that progress—not perfection—builds confidence.

Permit yourself to do well enough and still have time to rest. It's not settling—it's self-respect.

***

Creating a Flexible Routine

Routines help your brain feel calm, but they should serve you—not trap you.

Try color-coding your planner or digital calendar:

- **Blue** for schoolwork

- **Green** for sports or activities

- **Yellow** for rest and fun

When you look at your week, check whether any color is missing. If all you see is blue, it's time to add some yellow.

Schedule your downtime as intentionally as your classes. Block out movie nights, walks, art time, or journaling hours like appointments with yourself. Balance doesn't happen by accident—it's something you plan for.

And be flexible—swap activities when needed. Dropping an extra club for art class, saying no to another volunteer shift, or taking one fewer AP course doesn't make you less ambitious—it makes you wise about your limits. Your schedule should fit you, not the other way around.

***

Turning Study Sessions Into Something Sustainable

If long study marathons leave you drained, experiment with shorter bursts of focus. Break significant assignments into mini-blocks of time—20 or 25 minutes of work, then a short reward.

Your reward can be small but satisfying: a snack, a favorite song, or a few minutes of stretching. These pauses give your brain the oxygen it needs to keep going.

If you struggle to start, try the "five-minute rule." Promise yourself you'll begin for five minutes. Often, that's all it takes to find your rhythm.

You can also schedule friendship time like appointments—lunch catch-ups, study sessions, or walks after class. Relationships don't have to be squeezed in at the last minute; they deserve space on your calendar, too.

And don't underestimate rest. Short naps, quiet playlists, or guided breathing before bed all improve focus and energy. Sleep isn't wasted time—it's how your brain refuels.

***

The Fear of Saying No

Saying no can feel scary, especially if you're used to being the reliable one—the person who always helps, signs up, or says "yes" first. But every "yes" is a trade. When you say yes to everything, you're often saying no to yourself: no to rest, no to joy, no to peace.

Dropping something or setting a limit isn't quitting—it's choosing sustainability. You can't pour from an empty cup, and your value isn't measured by how much you do.

Think of it this way: creating space for rest doesn't shrink your life—it expands it.

***

Using Your Toolkit Your Way

You don't need to follow anyone's perfect system. Use the strategies in this chapter like a mix-and-match toolkit.

Pair the breathing exercises that calm you with the planning habits that work best for your brain. Combine visualization before tests with small rituals that ground you—like a cup of tea while studying or journaling before bed.

The goal isn't to copy someone else's version of balance. It's to design one that fits you—your personality, your schedule, and your limits.

When your life feels calmer, clearer, and more manageable, that's when you know you're doing it right.

***

Tiny Rituals That Ground You

Sometimes comfort hides in the smallest actions. If your nerves spike right before a test, try one of these sensory resets:

Draw a tiny star or smiley face in the corner of your test paper—it's a private reminder that you're capable.

Keep a smooth stone, bracelet, or lucky scrunchie nearby; rub it between your fingers as a tactile cue to breathe.

Under the desk, gently tense your fists for five seconds, then release. That tiny act releases muscle tension and recenters your focus.

These gestures might seem small, but they can pull your body out of panic and back into presence.

***

How to Say "I'm Overwhelmed" to Parents (Without Tears)

Sometimes the most challenging part of school stress isn't the test—it's the conversation at home. You want to do well, but you also feel like you're drowning.

Maybe you've noticed signs of burnout: snapping at family over small things, trouble sleeping, or a knot in your chest every time someone mentions grades. These are not weaknesses—they're warning lights.

Talking to your parents about feeling overwhelmed can feel scary. You might worry they'll be disappointed, dismissive, or say you're "just being dramatic." But keeping it all inside only builds pressure. The goal isn't to have a perfect conversation—it's to let them see you need help, not more pressure.

***

Start With Honesty and Specifics

Try starting with something direct but calm:

"I'm really struggling with school stress right now and need your help to figure it out."

"I'm trying to do my best, but it feels like too much. Can we talk about ways to make it easier?"

Being specific about what's hard helps them understand you're not just complaining—you're problem-solving.

If they interrupt or minimize your feelings, gently hold your ground:

"Can I finish? I need to get this out."

"I know it might not seem that big to you, but it's cumbersome for me right now."

Setting boundaries is a powerful way to show emotional maturity and self-respect. It's not about shutting people out, but about making sure your needs are met and your feelings are respected. It's a way to take control and feel less overwhelmed.

***

Make It Collaborative

Adults respond best when they see you're taking responsibility for your well-being. Instead of dropping a pile of problems in their lap, bring potential solutions.

You might say:

"I'm thinking about dropping one extracurricular for now so I can focus better."

"Could we set up a quiet hour after dinner where I can study without interruptions?"

"Would it be okay to take one day off screens this weekend to reset?"

You can even mention specific changes that could help—less screen time after 10 p.m., a mental health day when your schedule's packed, or shorter study sessions broken by walks or music breaks.

By prioritizing self-care and setting boundaries, you're showing that you value yourself and your well-being. This can help you feel less stressed and more in control of your life.

***

If Emotions Rise Mid-Conversation

Expressing your emotions openly can be a relief, even if it's a bit uncomfortable at first. It's a way to share your feelings and let others in, which can lighten your load and make you feel less alone.

Pause, breathe, and if needed, step away for a few minutes before returning to finish.

You can say, *"I need a minute, but I still want to keep talking."*

Letting your emotions show can actually help parents understand how deeply this matters to you. Vulnerability is not failure—it's honesty.

***

Reaching Out Beyond Home

If talking to your parents feels too hard right now, try another trusted adult—maybe a school counselor, teacher, coach, or youth leader. You could even start by writing an email or note instead of speaking face-to-face. Sometimes the words come easier on paper.

Many teens find comfort in opening up to a friend or sibling first—someone who "gets it" and can help you practice what to say. The important part is not staying silent.

Asking for help isn't giving up—it's giving yourself a chance to breathe again.

Journaling Prompt

- What signs show up in my body when I'm stressed?

- Who can I talk to when I feel overwhelmed?

- What's one small change that could make school pressure feel lighter this week?

Journaling helps your mind untangle what anxiety twists together. Putting your feelings on paper gives them shape—and once something has shape, it's easier to handle.

***

Final Reflection: Pressure Isn't a Personality

You're not your GPA, your test scores, or your productivity. Those things can change by the week—but your worth doesn't.

Tests measure what you know in a moment, not who you are. They don't measure kindness, creativity, resilience, or empathy—all the things that matter most.

Anxiety may still show up sometimes. But with every deep breath, every honest conversation, and every boundary you set, you're teaching your brain that you are safe, capable, and enough.

You don't have to earn calm—you can practice it.

You don't have to fight stress alone—you can reach for help.

And you don't have to prove your worth—it's already yours.

Your Time, Your Terms — Redefining What Busy Should Look Like

Being busy doesn't mean you're doing well—it just means you're doing a lot.

Embracing the relief of slowing down can be the most productive thing you experience. It's not about doing less, but about doing what matters most.

Your worth is not tied to a packed calendar or a color-coded planner. You don't owe anyone that.

Your schedule should reflect what fills you, not what drains you.

Some weeks, that might look like getting everything done; other weeks, it might mean protecting your peace, saying no, or resting without guilt.

When you start measuring your days by how grounded you feel—not how many boxes you checked—you take back control of your time, your energy, and your joy.

That's not laziness. It's wisdom.

You deserve a life that feels balanced, not just busy. It's not about doing more, but about doing what matters most.

***

Wrapping Up This Chapter

Finding balance isn't about doing more—it's about doing what matters. It's learning to notice when you're stretched thin and permitting yourself to pause.

Some weeks will overflow with plans; others will call for extra rest. This rhythm is not a sign of failure, but a part of your growth journey.

Listen to your body. Notice when you're running on empty. Learn to say no without guilt and yes without fear.

Because when you take back your time—on your terms—you don't just manage your life better. You live it more fully.

Up next: practical steps to build absolute confidence and own it—even when everything else feels shaky. These steps will include setting clear boundaries, learning to say no, and prioritizing self-care.

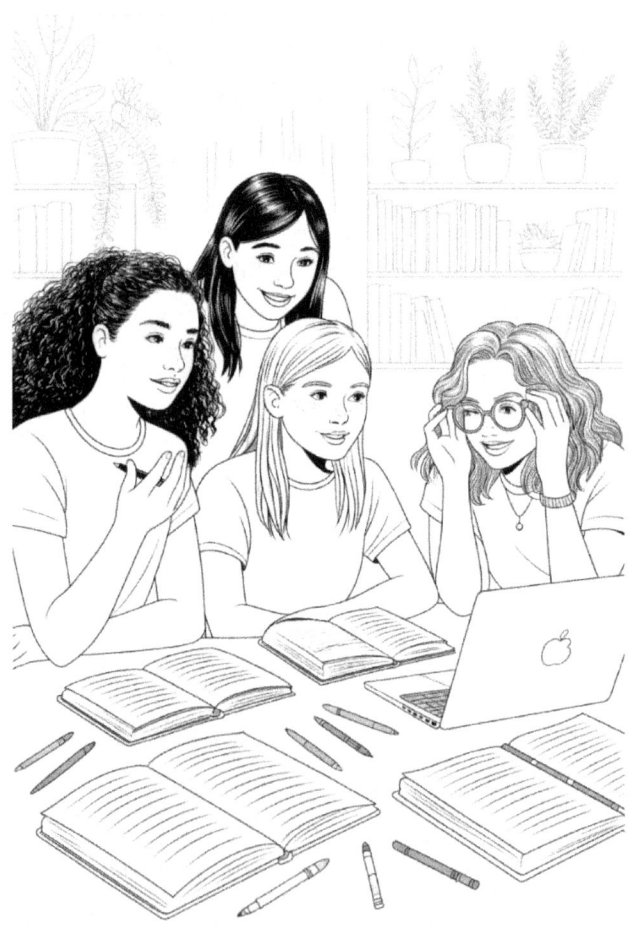

Chapter 5

Main Character Energy

Building Real Confidence (Not Just Faking It)

P icture this: you're standing at the bathroom mirror, toothbrush in hand, when it hits you—you actually messaged your teacher a question today instead of overthinking it. Or you walked past a group you usually avoid and looked up instead of staring at your phone.

These seemingly insignificant moments—**micro-wins**—are not to be underestimated. They are the tangible proof of your growth. They're not flashy movie scenes or social media highlights; they're the everyday choices that accumulate into something formidable. They don't need an audience to validate their importance.

Micro-wins are the steady heartbeat of absolute confidence.

***

WHY SMALL WINS MATTER SO MUCH

Perfectionism and self-doubt like to tell you that only big wins count—the lead role in the school play, the perfect test score, the viral post. When those things don't happen, your inner critic whispers, *"See? You're not enough."*

But that's a lie. Absolute confidence doesn't come from rare, shining moments—it's built from the dozens of quiet ones that nobody else sees.

Every time you do something brave or responsible, no matter how small, your brain gets a little reward—a chemical called dopamine. Scientists have found that your brain reacts to small successes much the same way it does to big ones. So yes, even something as simple as turning in an assignment on time or remembering to hydrate gives your brain a mini confidence boost.

Those moments train your mind to expect progress and to notice it. Each tiny action rewires your brain's "default mode" from *self-criticism* to *self-trust*. Over time, that pattern becomes your confidence foundation—not built overnight, but layered day by day.

***

Spotting the Micro-Wins You Already Have

Think about your week.

Did you get out of bed on a hard morning?

Speak up when something bothers you?

Finish an assignment early—or at least start one you'd been putting off?

Those count.

Confidence isn't about being fearless; it's about noticing when you act despite fear.

The truth is, you've probably already stacked up dozens of wins—you just haven't stopped to notice them.

How Micro-Wins Rewire Your Thinking

Here's the magic of acknowledging these moments: the more you identify small wins, the more your brain automatically seeks them out.

It's like turning on a light in a room you thought was dark. Suddenly, you see the proof that you're capable everywhere. You start replacing thoughts like *"I never finish anything"* with *"Actually, I started that project yesterday."*

Each time you record a win, you're reshaping your inner dialogue from *"not enough"* to *"getting stronger."*

***

Your Micro-Win Tracker

You can make this as creative or simple as you want—a journal, the notes app on your phone, a sticky note on your wall, or even a corner of your planner.

Draw seven boxes for the week or open a new note titled **"Micro-Wins."**

Each day, jot down one or two small victories.

Here's an example:

> **Micro-Win Tracker Example:**
> **Monday:** Asked for help in math — felt relieved and proud.
> **Tuesday:** Smiled at someone in the hallway — nervous, but accomplished.
> **Wednesday:** Finished an assignment early — less stressed.
> **Thursday:** Drank enough water — had more energy.
> **Friday:** Texted a friend first — brave and connected.

The details matter less than how the win *felt*. Confidence grows when you pause long enough to say, *"Hey, that was brave of me."*

Don't Underestimate Tiny Victories

Waiting for significant milestones—top grades, awards, recognition—teaches your brain to overlook progress in real time. But small wins are the roots of sustainable confidence. They're how growth actually happens.

One teen shared that her first micro-win was holding eye contact with her teacher during class. It felt awkward, but she did it. After a week of noting little moments like that, she realized she was speaking louder in group projects and laughing more freely around classmates.

Another reader decided to stop scrolling TikTok after midnight. At first, it felt like a silly goal. But two weeks later, she noticed her sleep had improved and her mornings felt calmer. Seeing that progress written down gave her motivation to keep going.

Confidence rarely arrives in one big moment—it sneaks in quietly, disguised as these small decisions you make every day.

***

Turning Micro-Wins Into a Habit

To keep your momentum going, end each week with a two-minute reflection. Ask yourself:

What did I handle better this week than last week?

Where did I speak up, even just a little?

What helped me feel calmer or stronger?

You'll start to notice that your answers expand over time.

And if you ever feel stuck, look back at your list. Seeing proof of steady progress—written in your own words—can instantly silence that inner critic whispering, *"You're not improving."*

***

The Ripple Effect of Sharing Wins

You don't have to keep your wins to yourself. Sharing them can amplify the joy and accountability.

Tell a friend about your best win of the week. You might inspire them to notice their own. Some teens even start a "micro-win" group chat where everyone posts one good thing that happened that day, no matter how small.

Families can do this, too—some make "win of the week" part of dinner conversation or write them on sticky notes for the fridge.

If saying it out loud feels awkward, keep your list private and reread it when you need a boost. Seeing how far you've come, even in small steps, can reignite motivation on the hardest days.

***

How Micro-Wins Transform Confidence

Over time, those small notes of progress accumulate. They become your personal highlight reel—one that isn't filtered, faked, or dependent on likes.

The more micro-wins you track, the louder your inner voice becomes—the kind that says, *"I can handle this."*

Significant achievements are a pile of tiny victories stacked together. Every new friendship, every time you spoke up, every morning you showed up when you wanted to hide—all of it counts.

Confidence isn't a lightning bolt—it's a slow sunrise.

***

Micro-Wins in Real Life

A few readers have shared how their lists changed them:

One wrote that after tracking daily wins for a month, she stopped apologizing so much. She realized she didn't need to prove she was "good enough constantly."

Another noticed that even when life felt chaotic, her list reminded her that progress was still happening. *"Seeing that list made me realize I'm not failing—I'm just growing quietly,"* she said.

Your list doesn't have to be fancy or perfect. It just needs to be *real*.

Your Challenge

For one week, track your micro-wins. Every day, write down one small thing you did that showed courage, effort, or kindness. It could be brushing your teeth on a hard morning, emailing a teacher, or putting your phone down when you need rest.

At the end of the week, read your list out loud. Notice how it feels. You might be surprised at how much strength is already there.

Confidence isn't something you wait to feel—it's something you *practice*.

***

A Final Reminder

Don't wait for someone else's approval to start seeing your progress.

Don't wait for a perfect moment to feel proud.

Every step, every attempt, every tiny act of courage builds a foundation of trust in yourself.

Absolute confidence doesn't shout—it grows quietly, beneath the surface, through all the little ways you keep showing up.

Keep noticing. Keep celebrating.

Because the main character in your story? She's already becoming stronger, one micro-win at a time.

***

HOW TO REFRAME "I'M NOT GOOD ENOUGH" THOUGHTS

That inner voice always seems to show up at the worst times—right before you raise your hand in class, try something new, or finally speak up.

It whispers things like, *"You're not smart enough,"* *"You don't belong,"* or *"You're going to mess this up."*

When those thoughts keep looping, it's easy to start comparing yourself to everyone around you. You might look at others and think, *"She's prettier."* *"They seem more confident."* *"Everyone else has it al have it all figured out."*

That voice—the one that lists everything you think you're not—is called **negative self-talk**. And here's the tricky part: it feels believable because your brain is wired to notice problems and threats faster than positives or praise. Psychologists call this a **negativity bias**. It's your brain's old survival system—great for spotting danger, terrible for building confidence.

The more you feed that bias, the louder the critic grows. But the moment you start noticing and naming those thoughts, you take back control.

***

Step One: Notice the Thought

The first step to quieting that inner critic isn't to argue or shove it away. It's worth **noting** it.

When you hear yourself thinking, *"I'm not enough,"* pause and label it. Literally say in your head, *"That's my inner critic talking."*

Then ask yourself a simple question:

"Is this a fact, or is this fear?"

Writing the thought down helps, too. Something about putting it on paper or typing it into your phone makes it smaller—something you can look *at*, instead of something that controls you.

***

Step Two: Catch It, Challenge It, Change It

Think of this as your three-step confidence reset:

Catch It

Notice when that self-critical voice pipes up. Pause long enough to name it:

"I just told myself I'm not good enough."

Naming the thought separates *you* from it—it's not your identity; it's just a momentary thought.

Challenge It

Ask yourself, *"Is that actually true?"*

Are you terrible at everything, or did you struggle once?

Would you ever tell a friend she's worthless because she made a mistake?

If not, why say it to yourself?

Your brain exaggerates failures and shrinks your successes. Challenge that habit by asking, *"What's the full story here?"*

Change It

Now rewrite the thought so it's **fair**, not fake.

Instead of *"I failed that quiz,"* try *"One quiz doesn't define me. I can review and do better next time."*

Instead of *"I'm not good enough,"* try *"I'm learning, and I'm proud of the effort I'm putting in."*

Instead of *"I'll embarrass myself,"* try *"It's brave to try, even when I'm scared."*

This isn't about pretending everything's fine. It's about speaking to yourself with honesty *and* compassion—the same way you'd talk to someone you love.

***

Building a List of Kinder Responses

Grab a piece of paper or your Notes app. Write down your most common "not enough" thoughts. Next to each, write a kinder, more accurate response.

Here are a few examples:

"I'm not smart enough." → *"I'm still learning, and that's how everyone grows."*

"I'm not pretty enough." → *"My worth isn't measured by my looks."*

"I don't fit in." → *"I'm still finding my people, and that's okay."*

The goal isn't to erase the first column—it's to balance it. Seeing both versions on paper reminds you that you get to choose which voice to believe.

At first, the kinder thoughts might feel awkward or forced. That's normal. You're retraining your brain. The more you practice, the more natural it becomes. Over time, supportive thoughts start to show up automatically.

***

USING AFFIRMATIONS THAT ACTUALLY WORK

Affirmations aren't about chanting empty lines in the mirror; they're about repeating truths your brain has trouble remembering.

Try simple statements like:

"I bring value just by being myself."

"I'm worthy of love, effort, and good things."

"I can learn new things, even if I mess up first."

Write them on sticky notes for your mirror, set them as your phone wallpaper, or tuck one in your planner. The more often you see them, the easier it becomes to replace self-criticism with calm reassurance.

Think of affirmations as gentle reminders—not loud pep talks. They're like small mental anchors that steady you when waves of doubt hit.

***

Give Yourself the Kindness You Give Others

Imagine your best friend said she felt ugly, stupid, or like she didn't belong. Would you list all the reasons she's right—or would you tell her everything you see that's amazing about her?

Give yourself that same grace.

You can even make it a mini writing exercise: write a short letter to yourself from the Perspective of that encouraging friend.

Start with, *"Hey, I know you're having a hard time, but here's what's still true about you..."*

Read it whenever you feel like you're slipping into old thought patterns. Hearing your own compassion in your own words can be one of the most potent ways to rebuild confidence.

***

Stories of Reframing in Real Life

One girl told me she convinced herself for years that she was "too shy" to audition for the school play. Each time, the thought *"I'll embarrass myself"* kept her frozen.

Finally, she decided to test the thought. She caught it, challenged it, and changed it to, *"It's brave to try, even if I'm nervous."*

She auditioned the next year—and got a minor role. Her goal wasn't perfection; it was proof that she could do hard things despite fear.

Another teen always called herself "awkward." She replayed every conversation, convinced everyone noticed her every stumble. One night, she wrote the phrase *"I'm always awkward"* in her journal and challenged it.

Was that really true? Did her friends avoid her, or did they laugh and stumble sometimes, too?

She realized everyone feels awkward—they hide it in different ways. That simple reframing helped her stop policing every word she said. Over time, she started speaking more freely and discovered she was actually pretty funny once she stopped overthinking.

Confidence didn't suddenly appear—it grew through honesty and practice.

Journaling Prompts for Reframing

You can use journaling to catch and reshape thoughts whenever they spiral. Try starting with one of these prompts:

- "A thought I have about myself that isn't true is..."

- "If I could give myself advice as a friend today, I'd say..."

- "One thing I did today that took courage was..."

Even a few lines can help shift your focus from fear to progress. The more you write, the clearer it becomes: your self-talk is just another skill you can improve with practice.

***

When Doubt Still Shows Up

Negative thoughts won't disappear forever—especially when you're under pressure or trying something new. Even the most confident people have moments of self-doubt. The difference is, they don't automatically believe those thoughts.

The goal isn't to silence your inner critic completely—it's to make peace with it. You can notice its voice, thank it for trying to protect you, and then gently remind it: *"I'm safe now. I've got this."*

You don't have to earn your worth or confidence—it's something you uncover as you grow.

***

Reframing Isn't Pretending—it's Perspective

Reframing isn't about slapping positivity over pain or pretending everything's perfect. It's about being honest and fair: seeing your strengths and your struggles, your mistakes and your growth, side by side.

Confidence isn't the absence of insecurity—it's the decision to keep showing up anyway.

So next time your inner critic speaks up, pause. Breathe. Ask yourself what's true.

You'll find that every time you rewrite a harsh thought into something kinder, you're not just changing words—you're building trust in yourself.

Give yourself the same compassion you so easily give others. You deserve it, every single day.

***

Main Character Energy Challenges — Owning Your Story at School

Having *primary character energy* isn't about being the loudest person in the room or having everyone's attention. It's about quietly owning your story—knowing that your experiences matter, your choices count, and your presence has impact, even when no one seems to notice.

It's not about perfection or popularity. It's about **belonging to yourself**.

Some days, you'll feel invisible, moving through the halls like an extra in someone else's story. Other days, you'll catch a spark—a reminder that you're capable of more than you think. That's your primary character energy trying to surface. It begins when you stop waiting for permission and start making small, intentional choices that align with who you really are.

Ask yourself:

"Do I speak up when something matters to me?"

"Do I try new things, even if I might fail?"

"Do I say no when I need to protect my peace?"

Every time the answer is yes—even in the smallest way—you're writing a stronger version of your story.

***

Small Challenges, Big Shifts

The main character's energy grows through small risks, not grand gestures. You don't need a dramatic glow-up or a viral moment to feel it. You need to keep showing up for yourself in little ways that build self-trust.

Start with **tiny challenges**—ones that stretch your comfort zone just enough to feel new.

It could be wearing something a little bolder or brighter than usual and noticing how it changes your confidence.

It could be introducing yourself to someone new in class.

It could be saying hi to the person who always eats alone.

The goal isn't to become fearless—it's to notice your courage *while you're still feeling the fear.*

Every small act of honesty, kindness, or bravery adds another line to your story—a story that's real, growing, and uniquely yours.

***

Track Your Growth in a "Main Character Journal"

Confidence builds when you see your own progress. That's where a **Main Character Journal** (or even a quick notes app list) comes in.

Each time you complete a challenge, jot down three things:

- What you did

- How you felt before and during

- How you felt afterward

You might notice a pattern—fear before, pride after. That's proof that bravery doesn't erase fear; it transforms it.

If something doesn't go perfectly, write about that too. What surprised you? What did you learn? How would you handle it differently next time?

Over time, these reflections become a living record of growth. You'll see how your confidence builds in layers, even when the results aren't visible yet.

***

Build Your Personal Highlight Reel

Think of your highlight reel as a celebration of courage, not perfection.

It doesn't have to be public or polished. You could save screenshots of encouraging messages, snap a selfie before a nerve-wracking event, or record a short voice memo describing how proud you felt after doing something hard.

If photos aren't your thing, keep a running list on your phone called **"My Main Character Moments."** Add to it weekly.

"Spoke up in class even though my voice shook."

"Tried out for something I've always wanted."

"Walked away from gossip."

"Helped someone without needing credit."

Each note becomes a scene in your story—a reminder that courage doesn't always look glamorous. Sometimes it seems like simply showing up when you could've stayed silent.

***

Celebrate With People Who Get It

Sharing your progress with someone you trust makes it feel more real.

Tell a friend, sibling, or cousin about something you did that scared you a little. Swap "main character moments" from your week—maybe one of you spoke up in a group project while the other set a boundary that used to feel impossible.

This isn't bragging. It's building a language of courage.

When you share your wins, you normalize growth—not perfection—and you make it easier for others to notice their own bravery, too.

***

What Growth Really Looks Like

Growth doesn't always give you fireworks. Sometimes, the reward is subtle.

Wearing that bold outfit helps you stand a little taller that day.

Trying out for a team leads to an unexpected friendship.

Walking away from a draining group chat might make breathing easier.

One student told me she joined the debate club even though she felt so nervous she was sick to her stomach. During her first meeting, her hands shook so hard she could barely hold her notes. But then she realized—everyone else was nervous, too. She walked out not just proud, but more herself.

That's what real primary character energy looks like: not spotlight confidence, but *quiet ownership of your story.*

***

Your Weekly Reflection: "How Did I Act Like the Main Character?"

At the end of each week, take a few minutes to write down your reflections:

"How did I act like the main character this week?"

Did you speak up for yourself? Walk away from a situation that didn't feel right? Try something that scared you?

Write about how those choices shifted your mood or self-image. You may have noticed less worry about what others think, or you may have felt a new sense of belonging.

The impact doesn't have to be huge to be real. Confidence often shows up quietly, in the way you carry yourself, the words you choose, and the people you gravitate toward.

***

The Heart of the Main Character Energy

The main character's energy isn't about outshining others or chasing constant attention. It's about **living intentionally**—making choices that reflect who you are becoming, rather than letting life happen on autopilot.

Every time you take up space, even briefly, you're reminding yourself:

"My story is worth telling."

You don't need an audience to matter. You need to keep showing up with honesty, kindness, and curiosity.

Over time, these small acts of courage build a story that feels truly yours—a life directed not by fear or comparison, but by growth.

Because the world doesn't need more copies of someone else's story.

It needs *you*—in all your messy, brave, imperfect brilliance—learning, laughing, trying, and rewriting scenes as you go.

So go ahead—take the pen back.

Be the lead in your own life.

Not because you're perfect.

But because you're real.

***

PRACTICING SELF-COMPASSION WHEN YOU MESS UP

Nobody likes messing up. Yet it's something everyone does—even the ones who seem to have it all together online. Mistakes, awkward moments, and disappointments are part of being human, not proof you've failed. Still, when something goes wrong, it's easy for that inner critic to grab the mic.

You might hear thoughts like:

"I'm such a failure."

"Why can't I ever get this right?"

"Everyone must think I'm so awkward."

That voice takes one mistake and stretches it into a story about your worth. Before you know it, your brain is replaying the moment over and over like a bad movie you can't stop watching.

But there's another voice available—one that's calm, fair, and gentle. That's the voice of **self-compassion.**

Self-compassion doesn't mean pretending everything's fine or brushing off responsibility. It means treating yourself the way you'd treat a friend who just messed up: with honesty, empathy, and perspective.

Instead of saying, *"I can't believe I said that in front of everyone; I'll never recover,"* you say, *"That was awkward, but I'm not the only person who's stumbled in public. People forget faster than I think. I'll be okay."*

One voice fuels shame.

The other fuels growth.

And here's the best part: research shows that being gentle with yourself after failure actually helps you recover faster and builds greater resilience.

***

Why Being Kind to Yourself Works

When you beat yourself up, your body stays in stress mode—your heart races, your stomach tightens, and your mind floods with "what ifs." But when you respond with compassion, your nervous system calms down. You literally help your brain and body shift from panic to peace.

It's not weakness; it's a reset.

Think of self-compassion as hitting the "pause" button on your inner critic. It gives you enough space to breathe, reflect, and try again without dragging guilt along for the ride.

***

Try a Simple "Breathe and Reset" Ritual

When embarrassment or regret hits hard—your cheeks flush, your mind spins, your heart thuds—stop and breathe.

> **Here's a quick way to ground yourself:**
> - Take a slow breath in through your nose for four counts.
>
> - Hold it for two.
>
> - Exhale slowly through your mouth for six.
>
> - Repeat this three times.
>
> As you breathe, imagine calm flowing in and tension flowing out.
> Then whisper to yourself:
> *"This doesn't define me. I'm allowed to make mistakes."*

It might feel awkward at first, but that single sentence creates space between you and the shame spiral. You're reminding your brain: *I can reset. I can move forward.*

***

Write a Forgiveness Letter to Yourself

Sometimes the guilt sticks around even after you breathe. When that happens, write it out.

Start a letter that begins with:

"I forgive myself for..."

List everything—big or small—that's weighing on your mind. Don't censor or judge it. Just let the words spill.

When you finish, read your letter as if someone you love had written it. Would you tell them they were unworthy? Or would you tell them they're doing their best?

Seeing your thoughts on paper helps relieve the emotional pressure that builds when regret stays trapped in your head. It's not about excusing mistakes—it's about making peace with your humanity.

***

Find the Lesson Hidden in the Cringe

Once the sting begins to fade, shift your focus from shame to learning. Ask yourself:

"What can this moment teach me?"

"What would I do differently next time?"

This turns the situation into a teaching moment rather than a punishment.

Maybe you froze during a class presentation and felt humiliated. Next time, you could practice out loud at home or record yourself to hear your pacing. You may have forgotten an assignment or misread instructions. Now you know you need a checklist or reminder system.

Mistakes are uncomfortable—but they're also information.

Then balance out your reflection by writing down **three things you did right**, even if the moment wasn't perfect.

Maybe you showed up even though you were nervous.

Maybe you apologized when you could've avoided the topic.

Maybe you finished what you started despite fear.

Focusing on what went right keeps your confidence alive, even in the middle of imperfection.

***

Real Stories, Real Recovery

One girl told me she forgot her lines during a class performance and wanted to disappear. Her voice shook, her face turned red, and she felt like everyone was staring. But she finished anyway.

When the next presentation came around, she remembered that moment—not as proof she wasn't good enough, but as evidence that she could survive embarrassment and keep going. Her confidence didn't come from being flawless; it came from not giving up.

Another teen said she snapped at her best friend after a rough week and instantly regretted it. Instead of ghosting or pretending it didn't happen, she took a breath, texted an apology, and explained she'd been stressed. That honest conversation didn't ruin the friendship—it strengthened it. Both walked away with a deeper understanding of each other.

These stories show what compassion in action looks like. It's not dramatic or perfect—it's brave, honest, and healing.

***

When Shame Starts to Spiral

Suppose you find yourself replaying a mistake again and again. In that case, it usually means your brain is trying to protect you from future embarrassment. It's like a misguided coach saying, *"If I remind you of this enough, you'll never mess up again."*

But shame doesn't teach; it traps.

When you catch yourself spiraling, say gently:

"I've learned what I needed from this. I'm allowed to move on."

Then redirect your attention to something grounding—step outside, stretch your shoulders, grab a glass of water, or focus on one comforting sound around you. These minor resets help your body and brain remember that the moment has passed.

***

Why Mistakes Don't Define You

Perfection isn't what earns you worth—being real does.

Think about the people you admire most. Chances are, they've all failed, messed up, or faced something embarrassing. What makes them inspiring isn't that they never stumbled; it's that they got back up, laughed about it later, and kept going.

The same is true for you.

Every time you practice kindness toward yourself after falling short, you're building emotional strength. That's what psychologists call **resilience**—the ability to bounce back, adapt, and keep trying.

You don't need to eliminate every mistake to be confident. You need to learn how to handle them with grace.

Journal Prompts for Healing After a Mistake

- *"A moment I wish I could redo—but can learn from—is..."*

- *"Three things I did well in that situation were..."*

- *"If my best friend were in my shoes, I'd tell her..."*

- *"One kind truth I can remind myself of right now is..."*

Answering even one of these helps transform guilt into growth.

***

From Shame to Self-Acceptance

Mistakes are unavoidable. But shame doesn't have to write the ending.

Self-compassion turns those moments that once made you shrink into stepping stones toward confidence. Each time you respond with gentleness instead of judgment, you're teaching your heart that it's safe to try again.

Remember: absolute confidence isn't built from perfection—it's built from how you treat yourself when things don't go as planned.

You can be both a work in progress *and* worthy right now.

***

A Final Reflection

When you stumble, take a breath.

When you cringe, smile softly at your own humanity.

When you fall, reach for grace before guilt.

Your story doesn't fall apart when you make mistakes—it deepens.

And every time you choose compassion over criticism, you turn the page toward strength.

Next up, we'll explore something many teens struggle with—**body image**—and how to see your worth far beyond the mirror. Because believing in yourself runs deeper than any awkward moment, grade, or misstep ever could.

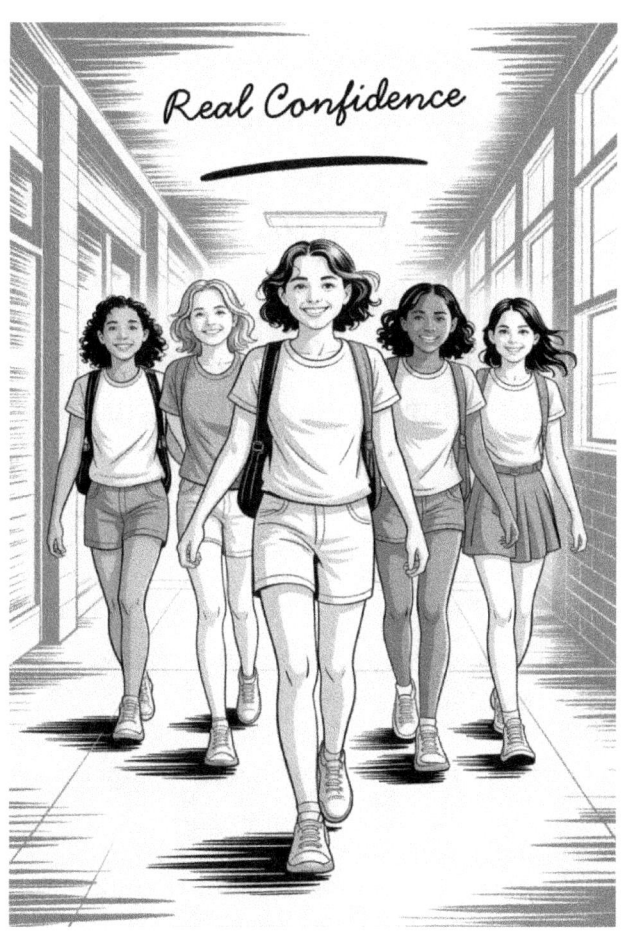

Chapter 6

Body Image & Media Myths

Seeing Yourself Beyond the Surface

When did you first *notice* your body?

It could be a random comment from a relative at a family dinner, or a comparison to a sibling or a friend.

It could have happened in gym class, changing under harsh fluorescent lights.

Or it was the first time you tried on an outfit that didn't fit the way you imagined.

For many of us, that moment of awareness arrives suddenly—like a spotlight shining on "flaws" we didn't even realize existed. Puberty only amplifies it. Our bodies change shape, our skin starts doing unpredictable things, and suddenly we're comparing ourselves to everyone around us. It can feel like we're living inside a body that doesn't quite belong to us anymore.

Friendships shift, too. You start hearing people comment on their own bodies—or each other's. Someone jokes about thighs or acne. Someone else posts about "glow-ups" or "summer bodies." Without realizing it, you begin scanning your reflection more critically, wondering if you measure up.

Even well-meaning family comments—"You've grown so fast!" or "You're filling out"—can echo in your mind for years. Words meant as observations sometimes land as judgment.

***

WHEN THE WORLD TELLS YOU TO CHANGE – REMEMBER WHO YOU ARE

Then there's social media.

Every scroll reveals a world of deception, with filtered faces, flat stomachs, poreless skin, and "perfect" angles—feeding the illusion of perfection.

Influencers talk about "self-love" while quietly selling products that promise to change you. Ads whisper the same message in a thousand different ways: *You'll be better once you fix yourself.*

You're shown an endless stream of "ideal" images—each one edited, posed, and polished. And after a while, it starts to work on you. You catch your reflection and think, *Why can't I look like that?*

But here's what the data says: more than half of teens, just like you, worry about their appearance, and nearly half of girls often feel dissatisfied with their bodies. That means if you've ever felt self-conscious, you're standing in a crowd—not alone.

The truth is, there's nothing wrong with wanting to feel confident in your own skin. What hurts is when the world convinces you that confidence only comes *after* you change.

***

Learning to Turn Down the Inner Critic

That critical voice in your head can get loud.

It says things you'd *never* say to your best friend.

"I'm gross."

"I'll never look right."

"I'm unfixable."

But you don't have to believe everything that voice says.

Thoughts are not facts—they're stories your brain tells when it's been fed too much comparison. To challenge these thoughts, you can try cognitive restructuring, such as replacing negative thoughts with more realistic, positive ones.

You can learn to turn that voice down and speak to yourself with fairness instead of judgment.

Start with a **body check-in.**

Stand in front of a mirror—not to inspect, but to notice.

See yourself as a whole person, not a collection of parts to critique.

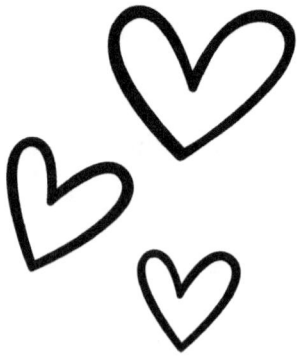

Then, name five things about yourself that have *nothing* to do with appearance.

Maybe:

- You can climb stairs without getting winded

- You make people laugh

- You have creative ideas

- You show up for your friends

- You're resilient

Write those on sticky notes and put them where you'll see them—on your mirror, notebook, or wall.

Say them out loud if you can:

"I am strong."
"I am loyal."
"I am creative."
"I am kind."
"I am enough."

These aren't empty affirmations—they're reminders of your *real* worth.

***

Respect Before "Body Love"

You don't have to adore every inch of your body to respect it. "Body positivity" can sometimes feel like pressure—like you're supposed to love your reflection 24/7 or else you're failing at self-acceptance.

The truth is, respect comes before love.

You can start with **body neutrality**—acknowledging your body as something that works for you, not against you.

Try a few grounded, honest affirmations like:

"My body is not an ornament; it's an instrument."

"I don't have to love everything I see to treat myself with care."

"My worth isn't measured in mirror angles."

Focus on what your body *does*—how it lets you dance, laugh, run, hug, breathe, create, or rest.

You don't need to fix your body to feel grateful for it.

***

Understanding Where the Pressure Comes From

When you find yourself wishing to change something—your skin, your legs, your height—pause before criticizing. Ask:

"Where did I learn that this is a problem?"

"Who benefits from me feeling insecure about this?"

Most of the time, the pressure doesn't come from your heart—it comes from marketing.

Billions of dollars are spent every year convincing people that they're "not enough," so they'll buy something that promises to fix it.

Recognizing that truth doesn't erase insecurity overnight, but it helps you separate **your voice** from the noise around you.

Journaling and Creative Reflection

If you can't find the right words, start with art instead of writing.

Draw or paint a self-portrait that celebrates what your body *does*.

Sketch your hands as they create.

Draw your legs like tree trunks—strong, steady, carrying you forward.

Use bright colors to show movement, laughter, and energy.

You might notice that by the end, your focus has shifted—from appearance to ability, from judgment to appreciation.

If writing helps more, try these prompts:
- *"How would I describe my body if it were my best friend's?"*

- *"What's something my body lets me do that I'm grateful for?"*

- *"What story am I telling about what I should look like—and do I actually believe it?"*

Even a few lines can shift your perspective from self-criticism to curiosity.

***

Small Stories, Big Shifts

One girl told me she spent years slouching after classmates teased her for being tall. She tried to make herself smaller in every room. Then one day, her coach told her, *"Do you realize how powerful you look when you stand up straight?"* It wasn't instant, but that moment changed something. She started walking taller—literally and emotionally.

Another girl said she used to call herself "gross" every time she looked in the mirror. Then she began noticing how her body let her dance for hours, carry groceries for her grandma, or stay up laughing with friends. She didn't suddenly love every part of herself, but she stopped calling herself names. That shift—from disgust to respect—changed everything.

Confidence doesn't always arrive with fireworks. Sometimes it grows slowly, through everyday choices: catching a harsh thought, standing straighter, or choosing clothes that feel like *you*, not what's trending.

***

Interactive Exercise: Mirror Talk Script

Try this simple daily ritual:

Stand in front of your mirror for one minute. Look at yourself—not to critique, but to connect.

Say out loud:
- *"I'm grateful my legs carry me every day."*

- *"My arms are strong enough to hold my favorite people."*

- *"My smile makes others feel welcome."*

- *"I am not just what I see—I am my ideas, my laughter, my courage."*

Do it once a day, morning or night, for a week.

You don't need to force positivity—just honesty.

You might notice, little by little, that your voice softens when you talk to yourself.

A Truth Worth Remembering

Your body is not the problem. The unrealistic standards around you are.

You are not a before-and-after picture.

You are not an algorithm.

You are not a filter, a number, or a trend.

Your body is your home—the place that carries your mind, your spirit, your laughter, and your ideas. It's the reason you can move through the world, experience friendship, and chase the things you love.

When you stop fighting your reflection and start listening to what your body's been trying to tell you—that it's tired, hungry, strong, or capable—you begin to build trust with yourself again.

That trust is where absolute confidence lives.

And to build that trust, here's one more way to reconnect with your body through gratitude and compassion.

***

Creative Reflection: A Letter to My Body

Write a short letter starting with:

"Dear body, I'm sorry for the way I've spoken to you. Thank you for..."

List what you're grateful for—movement, energy, senses, even recovery from sickness or stress.

This simple letter can reconnect you with gratitude and release some of the tension built up over years of criticism.

You don't have to show it to anyone. The act of writing it is enough.

***

One Honest Reflection at a Time

When you start practicing mirror talk and rewriting the stories you tell about your body, something powerful happens: you stop treating confidence as a prize you earn after changing yourself. You start seeing it as something that grows through how you treat yourself *now*.

Negative self-image doesn't get to decide your story.

Every time you choose kindness over comparison, every time you notice strength instead of "flaws," you quiet the noise and make more room for peace.

You're not supposed to look like anyone else—you're supposed to *look like you*.

And that's enough.

***

MEDIA MYTH-BUSTING — SPOTTING UNREALISTIC STANDARDS ONLINE

When you scroll through Instagram, TikTok, or binge your favorite show, remember: you're not seeing reality—you're seeing *an edit of it*.

Photos are filtered, brightened, and cropped to perfection. Videos rely on angles, lighting, and poses designed to make skin glow and bodies look smaller. What seems like a spontaneous post is usually the best take after dozens of retakes, sometimes touched up with apps like Facetune or Photoshop. Even "before and after" pictures are often staged—different lighting, posture, and filters can create a transformation that isn't real.

And yet, when you compare yourself to those images, your brain doesn't see "edited"; it sees *better*.

It's easy to forget: almost nobody looks like those photos all the time. Real skin has texture. Real bodies come in all shapes and sizes. Real mornings involve messy hair, eye bags, and imperfect lighting.

Editing apps can erase blemishes, fake abs, and change bone structure in seconds. Seeing these perfect pictures again and again can make your reflection feel wrong—even when it's simply *real*.

***

Behind the Screen: What's Really Going On

The next time you scroll, try becoming a quiet detective. Ask questions before you let comparison take over:

"Was this image edited?"

"What's just outside the frame?"

"Is this post trying to sell something—an image, a product, or a lifestyle?"

"Does this make me feel inspired or pressured?"

Try mentally rewriting influencer captions.

"Woke up like this" becomes "Spent an hour setting up lighting and retouching this."

"Just casual vibes" becomes "Choose this angle because it hides what I don't like."

When you name what's happening, the illusion starts to lose its power.

You can even train your eye to spot editing: look for distorted walls, repeated patterns, shadows that don't line up, or overly smooth skin. If every picture from an account looks flawless, ask yourself—why? Life isn't flawless.

Challenge yourself to pick one post this week and rewrite the caption honestly. Doing that simple exercise helps your brain remember: you're not looking at truth—you're looking at *performance*.

***

The Problem of Representation

Here's another layer: most media still show only a narrow slice of what's considered "beautiful."

Magazines, ads, and popular shows often recycle the same body types, skin tones, and hair textures while leaving many others out. Models are still mostly thin, light-skinned, and airbrushed. The result? Millions of girls rarely see people who look like them celebrated.

When your reflection doesn't match what's constantly labeled "beautiful," it's easy to believe you need to change to belong.

But things *are* shifting. More creators and brands are breaking the mold—showing scars, stretch marks, acne, disabilities, natural curls, and genuine smiles.

One teen told me she used to feel invisible searching for YouTubers with her skin tone and body type. When she finally found creators who looked like her—people who shared their stories honestly, not ideally—something inside her relaxed. *"I realized,"* she said, *"I don't have to fit in when I can stand out for being real."*

Representation doesn't just show you what's possible. It permits you to see your own reflection with pride.

***

Curating Your Feed for Realness

Your feed is your space—you get to decide who earns a place in it.

If scrolling leaves you anxious or insecure, try this simple reset:

Unfollow three accounts that make you feel smaller.

Replace them with three that lift you or expand your view of beauty.

Follow artists, activists, athletes, or writers who post real life—not just polished perfection. Look for creators of color, body-neutral voices, or people who share about mental health and growth.

Body-positive and self-acceptance accounts can remind you that you're not alone. Seeing real, unfiltered people in your feed retrains your brain to recognize normal bodies and genuine happiness.

This isn't just about positivity; it's about **balance**. A diverse feed helps you understand that beauty comes in a thousand shapes, tones, and textures—and that none is the standard.

***

A One-Week Feed Challenge

Here's something to try:

Curate your feed for *authenticity* for just one week.

Mute or unfollow anyone who consistently makes you feel anxious or "less than." Add creators who talk about creativity, kindness, humor, or personal growth.

Then notice:

- Do you feel calmer when you scroll?

- Does your mood stay steady instead of sinking?

- Are you inspired by ideas instead of appearance?

Screens reflect what you choose to see.

When your feed starts reflecting realness, your mind begins to relax—and your confidence grows quietly in the background.

***

Seeing Through the Myths

Understanding how the media works doesn't mean you stop enjoying it. You can still love fashion, photography, or influencers—but now you can enjoy them consciously.

Once you know a post is curated or monetized, you get to decide whether to take it seriously or appreciate it as entertainment.

Remember: online perfection is a story designed to sell *something*—products, attention, validation. It's not a standard for your worth.

When you stop comparing your whole, messy, beautiful life to someone else's edited feed, you free yourself from an impossible race you were never meant to run.

DRESSING FOR YOU, NOT THE ALGORITHM

Some mornings, the closet feels like a test.

Do you wear the yellow shirt that makes you feel happy—or the outfit that'll photograph well?

Trends move fast, and it's tempting to dress for likes instead of comfort. You could have saved styles that look perfect online but feel awkward in real life. Dressing for the algorithm might get you compliments, but it also makes you feel like you're wearing someone else's identity.

Absolute confidence doesn't come from what others approve—it comes from what feels *true*.

Clothes are tools for self-expression, not comparison. They can lift your mood, boost your confidence, and reflect your story without needing to fit a trend.

Think about the colors, fabrics, or shapes that make you feel grounded. It could be a soft hoodie, a bold print, or your favorite worn-in jeans. Notice what outfits help you stand taller or breathe easier.

Start documenting them—snap a mirror pic or jot a list in your Notes app. Those are your **confidence outfits**, not because they're stylish, but because they feel like *you*.

***

The Freedom to Be Unfiltered

The pressure to be "camera-ready" can drain the fun out of fashion.

Maybe you've worn painful shoes just for a photo.

Or copied a layered influencer look only to feel uncomfortable all day.

One girl told me she used to hide her favorite oversized sweater because it wasn't trendy. Then one day she wore it anyway—and got more genuine compliments than she expected. *"I felt so comfortable,"* she said. *"It was like everyone finally saw me for me."*

That's what authenticity does—it attracts the right kind of attention, not the kind that drains you.

***

Building a Confidence-Boosting Closet

You don't need a shopping spree to feel good in your clothes. Start with what you already have:

- **Do a closet reset**

Keep what makes you feel confident.

Donate what doesn't fit or drains your energy.

Re-style "maybe" pieces—sometimes a new combo brings them back to life.

- **Focus on comfort and authenticity**

Choose fabrics you love, not ones that photograph best.

- **Drop the rules.**

Ignore size labels and brand names. Focus on how something feels when you move, sit, or laugh in it.

- **Experiment**

Play with accessories, layers, and colors that spark joy. You're allowed to change your mind, evolve, and reinvent your look.

Fashion is supposed to be fun—a creative expression, not an audition.

***

Closing Reflection: Reclaiming Your Real

When you understand how much of what you see online is edited, staged, or filtered, something inside you softens.

You stop looking for flaws in the mirror and start questioning the myths instead.

Beauty stops being a race to the "ideal" and becomes a reflection of truth—your truth.

Curating your feed for authenticity, dressing for yourself, and remembering that media tells *stories*, not *facts*, help you return to your real life—where laughter isn't filtered and your worth isn't up for debate.

Your body, your style, your face—they're already telling a story.

Make sure it's *your* story, not the one the algorithm wrote for you.

Because the most powerful kind of beauty isn't the kind that trends—it's the kind that stays real.

***

MOOD BOARDS & INSPIRATION — DISCOVERING WHAT STYLE FEELS LIKE YOU

A mood board is one of the easiest ways to explore who you are through style—without pressure or perfection.

You can make one on paper with magazine clippings or on your phone using screenshots and saved posts. Collect outfit photos, colors, patterns, accessories, or even textures that catch your eye. Don't just copy influencers—look everywhere.

Movies. Street art. Nature. Music videos. The girl at the coffee shop whose outfit works.

As you gather, you'll start to notice patterns: maybe you're drawn to soft pastels and flowy fabrics, or bold prints and chunky boots, or a sleek monochrome vibe. Those recurring themes are little clues about your authentic aesthetic.

The goal isn't to become someone new—it's to recognize what you already love.

That awareness makes shopping and dressing less stressful. You'll buy fewer "trendy" pieces you never wear and more items that actually feel like you.

Your mood board becomes a mirror for your taste, not the internet's trends.

Try this: once your board feels full, scroll through it and ask, *What do these images say about me?* Confident? Playful? Calm? Artistic? Let those answers guide how you show up—not just in clothes, but in energy.

***

Thrifting & Experimentation — Dressing Without the Rules

Thrifting with friends is one of the most thrilling ways to experiment—budget-friendly, eco-friendly, and pure fun. It's like going on a treasure hunt, but the treasure is a unique piece that fits your style perfectly.

Unlike big-box stores, where every rack screams the same trends, thrift shops are full of surprises. You might find a vintage denim jacket that fits like it was made for you, a weird T-shirt that makes people smile, or a bold piece you'd never see online.

Each find has a story—and that story becomes part of yours.

One teen told me she used to copy influencer outfits just to fit in, but it always felt off. Then she started thrifting every weekend, mixing unique finds with pieces she already loved. Over time, her wardrobe turned into a reflection of her creativity. *"I stopped worrying about likes,"* she said. *"Now when people compliment my style, I know they're complimenting me."*

Experimentation builds confidence. When you take small risks with fashion—trying a new color, pattern, or silhouette—you remind yourself you're allowed to change and explore.

***

Authentic Connections — Style That Speaks Without Words

Here's the thing about authenticity: it's magnetic.

When you wear what feels right, you carry yourself with a newfound confidence. You stand taller, move more easily, and seem more approachable. And that energy attracts people who appreciate you for who you are, not who you're trying to be.

You might start getting compliments from unexpected places or notice how conversations flow more easily when you're comfortable in your skin. One girl told me, *"When I stopped dressing for what I thought people wanted to see, I started meeting people who liked the same music, the same art—it's like we recognized each other instantly."*

Your clothes can become quiet confidence cues. They say, *I know myself. I'm not trying to be someone else.*

You don't have to be loud to be seen—just genuine.

Small Experiments — Learning What Feels Like You

You don't need to overhaul your wardrobe to find your style. Just start with one small experiment this week.

Wear an outfit that makes you smile, even if it's not "on trend."

Add something bold—a pair of bright socks, a fun necklace, or a hat you've been too shy to wear.

Try layering differently or mixing patterns just because you can.

Then pay attention to how you feel throughout the day. Energized? Calm? More like yourself?

Keep track of what lifts your mood. Start a private Pinterest board, a phone note, or even a mini journal titled *"What Makes Me Feel Good."* Snap mirror selfies—not for posting, but to remind yourself of moments you felt confident.

Over time, you'll notice patterns—the textures, shapes, and colors that bring out your best energy. That's your *authentic style,* not something dictated by an algorithm.

***

Fashion as Play, Not Pressure

Somewhere along the way, fashion got tangled up with judgment. But it's supposed to be *fun.*

You don't need to follow every micro-trend or buy new clothes every season. You don't even need a "signature look." What you wear can shift with your mood, your growth, or even the weather—and that's the beauty of it. Fashion is your canvas, and you're the artist.

Try seeing your closet as an art studio instead of a battlefield. Mix pieces that don't "match." Re-wear favorites as often as you want. Play.

If something doesn't work, laugh it off—creativity is supposed to include trial and error.

Your style will evolve, just as you do. And as it does, your confidence grows quietly in the background—because you're no longer chasing approval. You're learning yourself.

Reflective Exercise: My Style Story

Grab your notebook or Notes app and write:

- *"When I feel most like myself, I'm wearing..."*

Describe the outfit, the colors, the vibe. Where are you? What are you doing? Who are you with?

Then ask:

- What about that look makes me feel grounded or joyful?

- How can I bring a piece of that feeling into every day?

This reflection helps you connect emotion to style—because true fashion confidence doesn't come from what's trending; it comes from what feels like *home*.

***

A Final Note: Fashion as a Mirror, Not a Mask

Fashion shouldn't cost your comfort, your confidence, or your authenticity.

The clothes you choose tell a story—but it's your story, not one written for likes or approval.

Each time you pick something that feels right to you, you're reminding yourself that you matter exactly as you are.

And the best part?

You'll start drawing people, opportunities, and moments that match that energy—because real always recognizes real.

***

GROUP SELFIES & COMPARISON TRAPS

You know that moment when someone says, *"Let's take a pic!"* and your stomach does a little flip?

Suddenly, you're wondering where to stand, which side of your face looks best, whether your smile feels forced, or if you even belong in the frame. Everyone's adjusting hair, tilting heads, chasing the "perfect angle."

And before you know it, you're comparing—faces, outfits, confidence levels.

You think, *She looks fantastic. Why do I look so awkward?*

Knowing the photo might end up online makes those thoughts louder. Filters and cropping can change everything—and sometimes it's hard not to wonder if you should've skipped the photo altogether. That's a lot of pressure for what's supposed to be a simple memory.

***

The Photo Pressure Loop

That quiet pressure shows up almost everywhere: lunch tables, team hangouts, birthday parties.

Even fun moments can start to feel like mini photo shoots. The goal shifts from *having fun together* to *looking fun together*.

But the truth?

The pictures that mean the most later are the ones that *aren't* perfect. The blurry laugh. The unposed hug. The photo where half the group's eyes are closed.

Those are the snapshots that tell the real story—not how flawless you looked, but how it *felt* to be there.

If retaking photos over and over stresses you out, it's okay to speak up. You can say something as simple as,

"I'm good with this one—let's just enjoy the moment."

Or,

"Let's do a silly one next!"

It keeps things light and reminds everyone that memories matter more than angles.

***

Locker Room Feels

Then there are locker rooms—another setting where self-consciousness can sneak up fast.

Changing around others can make you hyper-aware of your body in ways you wish it wouldn't. Maybe it's scars, stretch marks, or the way your stomach looks when you sit down. Even casual comments—"You're so skinny" or "I wish I had your legs"—can linger in your mind longer than anyone realizes.

Some girls seem totally relaxed, laughing or chatting easily, which can make you feel even more out of place. But here's the truth: *almost everyone feels awkward sometimes.* Some are just better at hiding it.

It's normal to want privacy.

It's okay to take your time or use earbuds while you change.

It's okay to stay close to a friend who helps you feel safe.

You don't owe anyone a conversation or explanation in that space.

If someone makes comments that make you uncomfortable, you can stay quiet or change the subject. You don't have to join in or respond. Protecting your comfort isn't rude—it's healthy.

***

Dressing Rooms & Shopping Trips

Even hanging out with friends can become an invisible competition.

You're in a cramped dressing room, your friend tries something on that fits perfectly, and everyone gasps, *"That's SO cute on you!"* Meanwhile, you're fighting with a zipper or staring at the mirror, comparing every inch.

It's easy to let those thoughts spiral:

Why can't I look like that? Why is this so hard for me?

But here's something to remember—clothes aren't emotional truth-tellers. They fit differently on everyone because bodies are different. Mirrors don't capture confidence, laughter, or kindness.

A little comparison is standard, but too much can drain you. When that happens, pause and ground yourself with this question:

"What's one thing I appreciate about myself right now?"

It could be your humor, your resilience, your kindness, or how you made someone's day better.

It's powerful to redirect your attention to something you *can* feel proud of.

***

Grounding in Realness

When comparison sneaks in, try this mini grounding tool:

Take a breath.

Name one physical thing you like (even something small—your eyes, your freckles, your smile).

Then name one *non-physical* thing you value about yourself.

The second one usually shifts your perspective faster.

Ask yourself: *If my best friend were standing here, would she point out my flaws or remind me of what makes me awesome?*

That's the voice to listen to.

***

How Others Broke the Comparison Cycle

Sometimes the best inspiration comes from real girls who've been there.

One high school basketball team started a tradition called "No Filter Fridays." After practice, they'd snap quick, unedited locker-room selfies—sweaty, messy, laughing. At first, it felt awkward. But soon everyone realized those photos showed something better than perfection: *real friendship.*

One girl shared that she used to hate group photos because she'd zoom in and critique her face every time. Then she started journaling after each photo day—writing what she noticed, what memories it held, and how it actually felt to be part of the moment. Eventually, she said, "I stopped worrying about how I looked. I started remembering how much fun we had instead."

***

Words That Help in the Moment

Having a few phrases ready can help you set boundaries kindly when things get uncomfortable.

Try these when needed:

"Hey, can we talk about something else?" — if the conversation turns into body talk.

"We all have different bodies—let's find what feels good for each of us." — when comparisons start.

"I'll sit this one out—catch me next time!" — if you don't want to be in a photo.

You don't need to explain or defend your choice. Short, calm responses are enough.

Your comfort matters more than the perfect picture.

***

Reframing Group Moments

You can't stop every comparison thought, but you *can* decide what to focus on.

When a group photo or locker-room moment makes you feel uneasy, remind yourself:

"This isn't about how I look—it's about the memory I'm making."

Later, when you look back, you'll remember the inside jokes, the laughter, and the chaos—not whether your hair was frizzy.

Try this journaling prompt afterward:

"What did I enjoy about this moment before I started comparing?"

That simple question can shift your brain from judgment back to joy.

***

Taking Back Power from the Spiral

Comparison thrives on silence and shame—it grows stronger the more you believe you're the only one feeling it. But here's the secret: *every girl in that photo has doubts.* Even the one who seems most confident is probably zooming in later, overanalyzing something about herself.

The next time you catch your mind spiraling, pause.

Take a breath.

And tell yourself:

"Everyone here is human. I belong in this picture just as much as anyone else."

That truth is your anchor.

Journal Prompts for Reflection

- *"What situations trigger my comparison thoughts most often?"*

- *"How do I want to feel in those moments instead?"*

- *"Who in my life helps me feel comfortable in my skin?"*

- *"What's one way I can make group moments more fun and less stressful?"*

Even jotting a few sentences helps you see patterns—and spot the people or spaces that actually support your confidence.

***

The Bigger Picture

Comparison in groups is standard—but it doesn't have to run your day. Every time you interrupt the spiral or change the subject, you take back a little power.

Remember: the most confident people you know aren't the ones who look perfect in every photo—they're the ones who can laugh off the imperfect ones and stay present.

Every girl you see, no matter how confident she seems, has her own moments of self-doubt. That's part of being human.

Confidence doesn't mean loving every photo or every reflection. It means remembering that you are more than what's captured in a snapshot.

Be patient with yourself.

Be kind to yourself.

Because absolute confidence grows in the quiet spaces where kindness replaces perfection and authenticity replaces comparison.

***

Looking Ahead

Being gentle with yourself is hardest when you're surrounded by mirrors, cameras, and constant comparison—but that's also when it matters most.

You're learning how to stay grounded in a world that keeps asking you to perform. That's real strength.

Next, we'll step deeper into the emotional space you've started to build—how to care for your mind and heart when stress builds up, expectations pile on, and you're not sure how to keep going.

Because confidence is just one piece of what it means to feel whole. The rest? That's what Book 2 is all about—finding your voice, setting boundaries, and living with purpose, from the inside out.

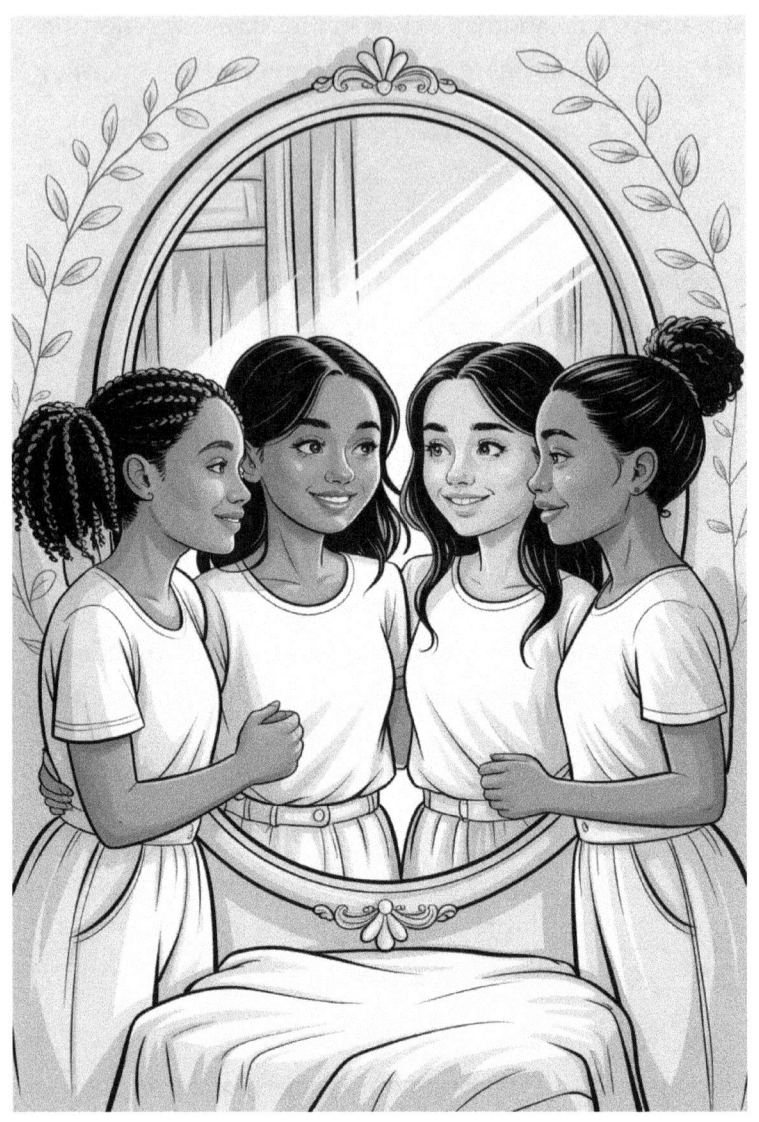

Conclusion

Before you close this book, I want one truth to settle in: **you are already enough.**

You deserve love, respect, and belonging—not because of how you look, how many friends you have, or how perfect everything seems online, but simply because you are *you*.

It's easy to forget that in a world full of pressure and comparison. But please remember: you don't have to shrink, edit, or change yourself to earn a seat at the table. You matter—precisely as you are.

We've covered a lot together. If you ever feel lost, flip back to any chapter and let it speak to you again.

We began by naming those lonely moments—the sting of being left out and the ache of watching life happen around you.

We talked about friendship: the joy of real connection, the confusion of drama, the lessons that come from forgiveness and trust.

We faced social-media pressure head-on and learned how to protect our peace in a world that rewards perfection.

We tackled school stress with fundamental tools—breaking tasks into steps, hitting reset after a hard day, and asking for help without guilt.

And we explored what confidence truly means: not perfection, but small, brave moments that build strength over time.

You also challenged beauty myths, learned to see your body with compassion, and practiced giving yourself grace when things felt heavy.

Each skill, each reflection, each tiny act of kindness toward yourself adds up to something powerful—**self-respect.**

By now, you've built a real-life toolkit for:
- handling friendship ups and downs
- managing stress and screens
- caring for your mind and body
- and building confidence that lasts

The biggest lesson? Change doesn't happen all at once.

It grows from small, steady actions—saying hi to someone new, choosing rest over pressure, speaking kindly to yourself when things go wrong. These micro-wins create absolute, lasting confidence.

Progress will never be perfect, and that's okay.

Keep journaling, reflecting, and giving yourself room to grow. If you stumble or slip backward, meet yourself with kindness—the same way you'd comfort a friend.

Your story is yours. There's no single way to be a teen girl. Your quirks, dreams, and doubts make your life one of a kind. **The world needs every kind of girl—quiet thinkers, loud leaders, creative dreamers, and everything in between.**

Celebrate what makes you different. Use what you've learned to lift others—to be the friend who includes, the person who listens, the one who makes others feel seen. Every act of kindness you offer ripples farther than you'll ever know.

Here's your next tiny challenge: choose one thing from this book and do it today.

Reach out to someone, set one small boundary, or start a mini goal just for you. Don't wait for perfect timing—every step counts.

As you move forward, hold this truth close:

You are seen. You are valued. You are never alone, even when it feels that way. Your worth is immeasurable, and the world is a better place with you in it.

I believe in your strength, your heart, and your ability to shape your own story. You have the power to overcome any obstacle and achieve your dreams.

Thank you for letting me be part of your journey. I'm cheering you on—**always**. You have a support system that will always be there for you, no matter what.

Stand tall. Own who you are. Keep shining, even when it's hard.

And when you're ready, Book 2 is waiting—to help you find your voice, set your boundaries, and keep growing into the person you were always meant to be.

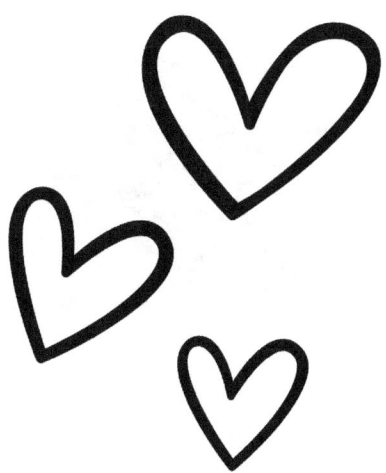

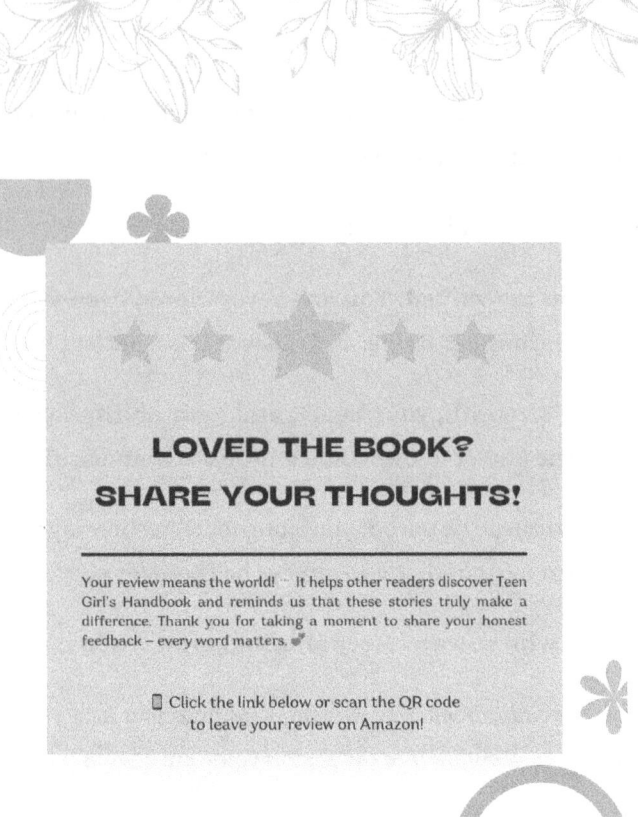

LOVED THE BOOK?
SHARE YOUR THOUGHTS!

Your review means the world! ~ It helps other readers discover Teen Girl's Handbook and reminds us that these stories truly make a difference. Thank you for taking a moment to share your honest feedback – every word matters. 💕

📱 Click the link below or scan the QR code
to leave your review on Amazon!

Scan the QR code to leave your review.

References

Talking With Your Child About Being Left Out
https://www.psychologytoday.com/us/blog/alone-together/202305/talking-with-your-child-about-being-left-out

Chapter 4: Social Media and Friendships
https://www.pewresearch.org/internet/2015/08/06/chapter-4-social-media-and-friendships/

The Influence of Social Exclusion on High School Students ...
https://pmc.ncbi.nlm.nih.gov/articles/PMC10676663/

100 Journaling Prompts for Self-esteem and Confidence
https://www.trishblackwell.com/442-100-journaling-prompts-and-questions-to-boost-your-self-esteem-and-confidence/

How to Help Your Teen Manage Toxic Friendships
https://www.newportacademy.com/resources/empowering-teens/teen-toxic-friendships/

When Your Daughter Isn't Invited, Why Being Excluded Hurts
https://www.thebravegirlproject.com/blog/why-being-excluded-hurts-parent-strategies-for-supporting-teens

Teens, Social Media and Mental Health
https://www.pewresearch.org/internet/2025/04/22/teens-social-media-and-mental-health/

A Teen's Guide to Setting Healthy Boundaries in Friendships
https://www.kidstuffcounseling.com/2024/02/20/a-teens-guide-to-setting-healthy-boundaries-in-friendships/

Exploring the effect of social media on teen girls' mental ...
https://hsph.harvard.edu/news/exploring-the-effect-of-social-media-on-teen-girls-mental-health/

Empowering Your Feed: The Art Of Deliberate Social ...
https://www.forbes.com/sites/forbeseq/2024/02/23/empowering-your-feed-the-art-of-deliberate-social-media-curation/

Preventing Cyberbullying: Top Ten Tips for Teens
https://cyberbullying.org/preventing-cyberbullying-top-ten-tips-for-teens#:~:text=NEVER%20OPEN%20UNIDENTIFIED%20OR%20UNSOLICITED,Delete%20them%20without%20reading.

Digital Detox and Well-Being | Pediatrics
https://publications.aap.org/pediatrics/article/154/4/e2024066142/199412/Digital-Detox-and-Well-Being

Why Does My Teen Procrastinate?
https://www.psychologytoday.com/us/blog/emotionally-healthy-teens/202006/why-does-my-teen-procrastinate

Test Anxiety Strategies and Study Tips for Kids
https://childmind.org/article/tips-for-beating-test-anxiety/

How to help children and teens manage their stress
https://www.apa.org/topics/children/stress

Balancing School and Social Life: 3 Tips for Teen Girls
https://rootsrenewalranch.com/balancing-academics-and-social-life-tips-for-girls-to-balance-school-responsibilities-with-social-activities/

The Science of Micro-Wins: How Small Daily Achievements ...
https://ahead-app.com/blog/confidence/the-science-of-micro-wins-how-sm
all-daily-achievements-rewire-your-brain-for-confidence-20250106-204735

How Teens Can Practice Reframing Negative Thoughts
https://www.newportacademy.com/resources/mental-health/reframing-nega
tive-thoughts/

Why GenZs and Millennials are all about 'Main character ...
https://www.harpersbazaar.in/culture/story/why-genzs-and-millennials-are-
all-about-main-character-energyand-heres-how-to-channel-yours-565375-2
023-03-26

Self-compassion: pre-teens and teenagers
https://raisingchildren.net.au/teens/mental-health-physical-health/about-m
ental-health/self-compassion-teenagers

Body image in childhood
https://www.mentalhealth.org.uk/explore-mental-health/articles/body-imag
e-report-executive-summary/body-image-childhood

Snapchat filters changing young women's attitudes - PMC
https://pmc.ncbi.nlm.nih.gov/articles/PMC9577667/

13 Body Positive Instagram Accounts That Make Teens ...
https://grownandflown.com/13-body-positive-instagram-accounts-teens-feel
-great/

Self-Esteem Worksheets for Teens
https://www.therapistaid.com/therapy-worksheets/self-esteem/adolescents

How Anxiety Affects Teenagers
https://childmind.org/article/signs-of-anxiety-in-teenagers/

How to Talk About Mental Health - Young People
https://www.samhsa.gov/mental-health/what-is-mental-health/how-to-talk
/young-people

Real   Stories   On   Mental   Health   From   Young   People
https://www.youngminds.org.uk/young-person/blog/

99   HEALTHY   COPING   SKILLS
https://www.akronchildrens.org/files/99-Healthy-Coping-Skills.html

Social   Belonging   and   Confidence
https://mhanational.org/resources/social-belonging-and-confidence/

Navigating   Cultural   and   Spiritual   Identity   in   Multi-   ...
https://danieldashnawcouplestherapy.com/blog/navigating-cultural-and-spi
ritual-identity-in-teens

Resource Center https://www.thetrevorproject.org/resources/

5 Safe   Online   Communities   for   Teens   That   Parents   Can   Trust
https://www.brightcanary.io/online-communities-for-teens/

Assertiveness (for Teens) https://kidshealth.org/en/teens/assertive.html

Helping   your   teen   set   boundaries
https://www.loveisrespect.org/resources/helping-your-teen-set-boundaries/

Difficult   conversations   with   pre-teens   and   teenagers
https://raisingchildren.net.au/teens/communicating-relationships/tough-topi
cs/difficult-conversations-with-teens

How   To   Help   Kids   Navigate   BFFs   and   Conflict
https://lindastade.com/teenage-arguments-with-friends/

Diet,   Sleep,   and   Mental   Health: Insights   from   the   UK   ...
https://pmc.ncbi.nlm.nih.gov/articles/PMC8398967/

11 Self Care Ideas for Teens https://www.talkspace.com/blog/self-care-for-teens/

Creating   Your   Own   Adjustable   Self-Care   Toolkit
https://foundrybc.ca/stories/self-care-toolkit/

8 Symptoms of Teen Burnout and How to Prevent It
https://www.newportacademy.com/resources/mental-health/teen-burnout/

How to Teach Growth Mindset to Teens
https://biglifejournal.com/blogs/blog/teaching-teens-growth-mindset?srsltid
=AfmBOop-gsYkoUwu_w28aMNkG8LXOdaKxJxkfEVnVFevTnGVfpmSJSVu

Failing Forward: 7 Stories of Success Through Failure
https://breakingmuscle.com/failing-forward-7-stories-of-success-through-fai
lure/

How to Help Teens Set Effective Goals (Tips & Templates)
https://biglifejournal.com/blogs/blog/guide-effective-goal-setting-teens-tem
plate-worksheet?srsltid=AfmBOopyHoNIqqWdzX6xGmpm4dNyHcoltzC-ZF
Wi-_12eebpDAU1j_GA

Celebrating Progress, Not Perfection: A Guide for Parents of ...
https://www.genieeduhub.com/post/celebrating-progress-not-perfection-a-g
uide-for-parents-of-teens

What to Look for in Friendships: Pre-Adolescents and Teens
https://evolvetreatment.com/blog/tween-friendships/

Self-advocacy: helping teenagers speak up for themselves
https://raisingchildren.net.au/teens/development/social-emotional-develop
ment/self-advocacy-helping-teenagers-speak-up-for-themselves

Speaking up changes everything
https://confidentteens.co.uk/speaking-up-changes-everything/

Kids, Teens, and Young Adults
https://www.nami.org/kids-teens-and-young-adults/

www.ingramcontent.com/pod-product-compliance
Lightning Source LLC
Chambersburg PA
CBHW061759120626
46550CB00005B/2064